PRACTICALLY PAGAN

An Alternative Guide to Health & Well-being

PRACTICALLY PAGAN

AN ALTERNATIVE GUIDE TO HEALTH & WELL-BEING

Irisanya Moon

MOON BOOKS

Winchester, UK
Washington, USA

JOHN HUNT PUBLISHING

First published by Moon Books, 2020
Moon Books is an imprint of John Hunt Publishing Ltd., No. 3 East Street, Alresford
Hampshire SO24 9EE, UK
office@jhpbooks.net
www.johnhuntpublishing.com
www.moon-books.net

For distributor details and how to order please visit the 'Ordering' section on our website.

ISBN: 978 1 78904 377 8
978 1 78904 378 5 (ebook)
Library of Congress Control Number: 2019956961

A CIP catalogue record for this book is available from the British Library.

Design: Stuart Davies

UK: Printed and bound by CPI Group (UK) Ltd, Croydon, CR0 4YY
US: Printed and bound by Thomson-Shore, 7300 West Joy Road, Dexter, MI 48130

Contents

Acknowledgements

I offer thanks to the family from which I came, for all of their imperfections and all of their strengths. I offer gratitude to a mother who gave me tools of resilience, even from a young age. She offered practices of mindfulness and positive self-talk. She offered me the advice to always take care of my body first and that any bad day would end. I am grateful for these tools and the way they held me after her fatal accident.

I am grateful to the beauties in my life who remind me that health is more than uneventful trips to the doctor. I am grateful for those who have held me when I needed to be held and encouraged me to come back when I needed to come back.

I think of health and wellness as the changing of the seasons and the way that everything needs to become fallow sometimes. I think of the way we need more care and sometimes we just need to be left alone.

I am grateful for many beloveds who have supported me through a series of traumas. I remember one who reminded me that they would be my Ninshubur and would seek me out if I stayed in the underworld too long.

Thank you.

And of course, thanks to Trevor and the folks at Moon Books for believing in me and my writing. I have been challenged, blessed, and made more resilient in the process.

I thank the godds, my body, and Mystery. I thank the journey of coming back to myself, in all of its complexity, loss, and wonder.

Author Note

I am not a healthcare practitioner or mental health professional. The words and advice in this book are meant to be a guide for supporting your well-being and are not meant to take the place of physician, psychologist, or psychiatrist advice.

Please continue to take any and all medications that you might be prescribed, even if the exercises and advice in this book may help you feel more grounded and centered. If you are considering changing any of your current healthcare regimens, always speak with your doctor first.

This might be a time to make big changes, but you will want to have your entire healthcare team in the loop about what you're about to do. And let's get honest here. I am certainly not perfect in my practice of self-care. I consider myself a work in progress and a promise in motion.

Reader, please know that you do not have to be perfect to be healthy. You can show up in the way(s) that you do. All I ask is that you continue to believe you are worth showing up for because you are. You are wondrous and worthy of attention and celebration. I already celebrate you for arriving just as you are. Just as you are today.

Introduction

You are precious. Your body is precious. Your mind is precious. Your heart is precious. With your actions, with your connection to yourself, you create a foundation that can weather all that comes before you.

Perhaps you have been told otherwise. Perhaps you have believed otherwise, that somehow, some way, you are less than worthy of love and care. Perhaps you know you are worthy of love and care and beauty, but need to be reminded or given permission. I want to tell you that your health, your well-being is valuable. And the actions you take to care for your beautiful self are a gift and a sacred prayer of intention.

With each breath, with each choice you make, you can call back the parts of yourself that have wandered away from knowing health and wellness. With each step toward what you want to feel and be, you create a song of belonging fully to your power.

No matter how you identify and no matter what your beliefs might be (if only for this moment), you can step fully into the shape of your skin. You can fill up the spaces of your being and the stretch of your authentic self -- you can move fully into your life.

It doesn't matter to me if you've been lost or not. It doesn't matter to me if you've made mistakes or you've fallen away from a path. It doesn't matter to me, as Rumi says, if you've broken your promises a thousand times. You can begin again. You can commit again. You can arrive in this precious moment. For you are a precious moment.

Starting Where You Are / Getting to Know Your Body

Before you begin, I invite you to release all attachments to perfection. The overculture wants you to think that no matter what you do, it will never be enough. Society tells us that no matter what we do, there will always be someone better, there will always be something more that 'should' happen. Let it go.

There is no one answer or one direction. While a simple answer seems the ideal path, it is also a journey of disappointment. Let's release that. Let's transform the energy of expectation into the energy of trust. I invite you to trust your deepest knowing. I encourage you to believe that you can care for your body, mind, and spirit, even if you're not 100% sure what the next steps are.

As Glennon Doyle says, "Just do the Next Right Thing, one thing at a time." And to be clear, your right might not look like my right. You may need another right thing or another right step. You might also need a place to begin. I offer that beginning. I offer an invitation to start now.

How to Release Perfection

If you are holding onto any old stories or messages about being perfect, this is the time to set them free. You don't need them where you're going. You don't need them in this world you're recreating for yourself. You can let them go, let them fall to the side and step into something different.

When we can let go of perfection and the message that things should look a certain way, we can quiet our conditioning and listen to the truth of our bodies. The body has messages for us. The body has questions and concerns, to be sure, but it also offers wisdom.

We need to remember how to trust our body. We need to build a relationship with our body by getting to know where we are right now. For some, this might be a new idea and for others, it might be a reigniting of an old and possibly tattered relationship. Let's create a new groove in our thinking. Let's create a new pathway, open up a new door, and walk bravely through it. We can start by leaving our luggage at the landing.

Letting Go of the Old Stories

There are stories that follow us, no matter where we go and no matter where we've been. We have stories of things that we've done, things we haven't done, and things that have been done to us. All of these stories, remembered and not, have shaped us into who we are today.

While we may not have asked for the shaping and we may not have wanted the feelings they have etched on our bones, these stories are alive. The stories have made us think things about ourselves that we may not have thought without them.

Some stories conjure up bravery, while others might offer anxiety. You might be someone who has stories they have never told to anyone else, possibly because of their horror or their sadness or the deepest desire to hide them. These stories are important. They deserve time and attention. They have lessons to offer. They have weight and texture and they trace the lines of our bodies more than we may realize.

For the stories that ache in the heart, I invite the possibility you can release them and unburden yourself. They may not go away and as they are a part of you, they cannot leave entirely. But they can be a hazy truth and not an obstacle to your life.

Write it down, transform it

One of the common practices in trauma therapy is to tell your story over and over until it loses its charge. When you start to tell a story so many times that the emotions just become words, and the words become almost nonsensical when they're repeated, you begin to separate yourself from the story.

For some, however, this practice can also be upsetting and activating. I offer that you can also place the words on a piece of paper where they can separate from you even more. You might choose to write out the story that you want to release or you might type it out and print it. Whatever works for you.

You might choose to draw the story or the image that most comes up when you think of the story in your mind. You might sculpt it. You might think of another physical way to show the story in a way that brings it alive for you.

I suggest finding time when you can be alone for this important practice. You will want to have space to feel feelings that arise as you write and as you remember. Take the time the story takes to be birthed into a form that can be destroyed in some way.

- You might choose to write the story on an old plate with a permanent marker and then smash it to pieces.
- You may choose to write the story on a piece of paper, kiss it, and then burn it to ash.
- You might smash a clay sculpture.
- You might rip a piece of art to shreds.

Allow yourself to feel into the story deeply before you consciously destroy it. In truth, matter is never created or destroyed, it is only shifted into another form. That form can be the thing that releases you, absolves you, and restores you. Re-stories you.

The story you choose can be one that has the most potency and power for you today. Or you might choose several stories. You might choose a person or a place or a situation. You may choose to repeat this exercise a few times until you feel free. Or you might choose to release one story that has been holding you back the most. And perhaps you'll come back to another when it feels like it's time. You are in control about how this process might look and how often you return to it. In my experience, once one story is released, it becomes clear that there are other stories attached to it that need to be freed as well.

Rewrite the story

For those who might have a story that has played in their head over and over in their life, destroying might seem too easy -- or perhaps not the first step. If that feels right to you, you may want to opt for rewriting the story. You can do this by writing out what the story is to you, just the way you tell it to yourself. Look at this story and identify who the main characters are. Look at how they interact and what doesn't work for you in this moment.

What would the story look like if things were different? Would the characters have said different things? Would they have made different choices? Would they have been in the story at all?

A practice I find helpful when seeking to release stories of pain is to rewrite the story as though I were the hero of the story. I will often write the story as though I'm a fairy tale character that faces something difficult, but then figures out how to solve the problem. The character I become might use tools, weapons, or magic. All things are possible in this landscape.

The story doesn't have to be long, but you will want to resolve things. You will want to resolve the problem and allow yourself to emerge victorious in the end. If you're not interested in writing, you can also create a picture of yourself in the story that holds more power and more presence than you did in the actual timeline of events. You might place a crown on your head or a sword in your hand.

You will want to find a way to recreate the story so you are not a victim or a bystander. You can make it about 'she' or 'he' or 'they' if that suits you more than using your name. Or you might rename yourself to give yourself a powerful presence that knows how to face difficult things. The key of this exercise is to make sure you rewrite things so they are 'better' in the end, however you might define that.

Make a soundtrack

It can also help to sink into your story with music. You might use your favorite playlist system to create a soundtrack that empowers you. Since everyone has different versions of what this might look like, you will need to be your own guide here. Find songs that allow you to feel energized. Fill the playlist with words and instruments that move through your body and make you feel good. These need to be songs that instantly make you feel better, alive, in control.

Once you have those songs, bring the story that you want to change into your mind. Turn on the music and see how the story shifts as you bring in movement and sound. Perhaps you think of the story and sway in time with the music. Perhaps you act out the story in a new way because the music offers wisdom that your thinking brain can't access with that memory. Or maybe you just turn on this music whenever a story starts to rise in your mind and it nudges you into old patterns.

- Allow yourself to be lost to the music.
- Allow yourself to be lost in the waves of possibility.
- Allow your body to guide you towards memories and through the emotions that live there.

For those who resonate more with movement than with writing, this might be the first point of your journey of release. For some, you might need a soundtrack of sadness or anger to move through your story before you can shift to power. Let yourself know and trust and feel into your needs.

Find a sacred witness

In an ideal world, we would have people in our lives that would listen to us without judgment, without trying to fix or correct. In an ideal world, we would be able to call on someone to be a witness to our healing. If you have such a person or you think you have such a person, they can be an ally in this work you are doing. You might ask a person to sit with you as you share a story that you want to shift. You can ask them to simply listen until you are done and to not offer any insights or responses. You can ask them to hold space for you until you feel you are done. You might ask this person only to thank you for sharing the story, for trusting them enough to be a sacred witness.

You might offer how you want to shift the story and how it has held you back. Again, this person is asked to not respond or to give advice. Just be witnessed in where you are or where you've been -- without any words that might land as judgment.

If you don't have a person like this, you can also do this practice with a mirror. You can tell yourself the story and look yourself in the eyes to witness yourself. You can also tell your story to a sacred statue or to a pet. Again, allow yourself to be heard and witnessed. Let yourself be held in the way that you need to be held.

You might tell a tree. You might tell a flower. Whatever you do, whatever/whoever is a witness, be willing to let the story go through you and out of you.

Feel all the feelings

When you are releasing the need for perfection and other stories, you are likely to notice various feelings arrive. These feelings might be expected or they might surprise you, depending on the story's content and its power. You might move from anger to sadness to confusion and back again. You might feel happy instantly once you have been heard, but then get angry about not feeling heard in the past. This is all normal and expected. This is all part of the 'moving through' process.

I hesitate to say healing, as the stories are not necessarily problems. The stories you hold might be challenging and they may have an impact, but they are not signs you need to be fixed. The stories you hold are a part of who you are in this moment. In fact, in any of this journey together, I will hesitate to talk about fixing things or healing things. You are not a problem. You have never been a problem. You are a being with things that have happened to you, things that have been a part of your experience.

To have feelings is natural and expected. During this process of creating distance from stories that do not serve you as well anymore, you may have to spend some time feeling upset. Let others in your life know that you are doing some personal work and that you may need time to yourself (or you may need a pass in case you have a reaction that comes out of nowhere).

On the other hand, this doesn't mean you need to cry all the time in order to be doing good work. Allow yourself to feel what needs to be felt. Just as it is. Perfectly as you are. That said, emotions will often arise when we least expect them to arrive. There are feelings we didn't feel safe to feel in the moments when things happened.

Sometimes, the unraveling of stories will unleash the floodgates. Release it all. Feel the feelings. Thank them for making their presence known. Let them know they are safe now. They can come out and be witnessed. Once you have moved through feelings that need to be expressed, you may find new feelings take up their place. Joy. Contentment. Happiness. Relaxation. Calm.

How to Create a Direction and Intention

Just like any new road trip, if the destination is new, we may not know what roads to take. In this journey of discovery, we might not have satellite navigation or GPS, but we can create an intention. I work with intentions in rituals and spells, and they are easy to use in the work of health and well-being.

An intention is a simple phrase that reminds you of your core action. What do you want to do in this journey? What are you looking to shift, change, or invite? What is at stake as you take action steps toward something new? I will often begin to create intentions by writing out the words that make the most sense with what I'm trying to achieve. Or I might write out words that feel powerful to me:

Power
Strength
Health
Balance
Self-Care
Grounded
Wellness

It can help to work on finding this direction as soon as you can. While it doesn't have to be the only intention you ever create (and you can always shift things as you learn more about yourself), it is very helpful to begin somewhere.

- What is important to you right now?
- What is active for you right now?
- What do you want to bring into your life?

I suggest focusing on what you want to bring into your world vs. what you want to remove. We already did some work on removing, so that energy is already called into (and out of!) the space. Now, we want to activate the focus on what you DO want.

- What do you need?
- What do you really want?
- What do you want to create?

Take some time to think on all of these questions and the answers that sing to you. Ideally, you will want to create a one sentence intention or direction, as this will be easy to remember and easy to recite in your mind.

I call my health back to my body.
I am worthy of love and self-respect.
I am ready to activate my intuition.
I trust my body to tell me what she/he/they need.
I support my health and well-being with new habits.

Some will find they want to be more specific rather than hazy. This is great. And some will find they want to keep things open-ended until they know exactly what works for them. As with anything in this book, choose what works best for you.

What is important with intention setting is that you believe in what you write. Believe what you mean so you are bolstered by the intention and empowered. Each time you read this intention, you feel like you know your path and your direction. Other examples include:

I am a strong person who asks for what I want.
I nourish my body, mind, and spirit.
I am healthy and happy and safe and strong.

I encourage you to find a few intentions that settle well in your body. And if you can't land on just one, find a few and drop into the wisdom of your body. Read the intention and scan your body to see how it feels. Do you feel excited? Do you feel inspired? Do you feel eager?

If your body isn't energized by the intention, you may want to rework it or move on to another option. Check in with this intention every day. Say it to yourself, remind your body of what you promise to them, and consider how your choices align with your intention during the day.

Becoming Truly Present

Being present is a gift to yourself and to others around you. When you are able to be in this moment, you allow yourself to make the next best decision. You can push away any competing thoughts or distractions. You can drop into what you really need and want. There are a few ways to cultivate presence:

Meditation - Though there are many more resources for meditation, I'd like to share a simple meditation that works well for those who need to quiet their minds. What you want to do is start with coming to your breath. You don't need to breathe deeply and you don't need to focus so much on what your breath sounds like or whether it's coming from your nose or mouth. Just breathe. Breathe into your lungs and out. Focus on the fact that you are taking in oxygen and releasing carbon dioxide, focus on the fact that you are breathing with the air around you and the plants and the beings. And just continue to breathe until you stop being aware of how often you're breathing and if you're doing it right. Your mind may wander and this is just fine. Allow your awareness to come back to your breath. You don't have to be in a particular pose, though sitting is often easier as it keeps you from falling asleep. Repeat this exercise for as long as it takes until your mind settles. Then slowly bring yourself back into the physical location of your body. Repeat daily or as often as needed.

Nature time - If you're a person who prefers to move than to sit still, then head outside for a nature walk. All you need to do is to stay present to what the world looks like around you. Notice the leaves, the trees, the birds, the animals, and anything else that happens to be around you. If you're around people, notice them. Try not to have headphones or music since it allows you to be more present in the moment. Walk around until you are settled and grounded, or relaxed.

Gratitude - If you're a person who gets caught up in what's already happened and what's about to happen next, it can help to create a journal for gratitude. All you need to do is to write out a few things that you noticed and are grateful for in your life. Ideally, you will want to be as specific as possible to that day in which they happened. Some folks find it easier to write these gratitude statements down at night before bed to bring them back to the present day.

Being present is about being mindful, about recognizing what is happening NOW. When you can come back to the now, you can really know what your body needs. And while anticipating needs is good, when you focus less on the 'should,' you can arrive at a more authentic answer.

Using Creativity to Focus

Once you have released and transformed stories, created an intention, and found presence, you can further hone your focus. I find that I need multiple ways to align my mind and my energy with my actions.

Creativity can help us bypass the think-y brain that wants things to be pristine and orderly. It can help us access the child part of ourselves that does things because they feel good versus how they look to others. We can leverage creativity to access what we need for our growth and what we need personally to move ahead in the way we want to move in our lives.

Setting up an Altar of Support

No matter what your beliefs, an altar is a traditional way to focus your energy. By having a physical space that reminds you of what you want or what's important, you can come back to this place for reminders and energy.

You can create a space that reminds you of why you're doing something, how you want to feel, and what your goals are. An altar doesn't have to be complicated or expensive or even intrusive. It can be simply a collection of things that gather up your energy. You might create an altar with:

- Your intention written out
- A few things that make you feel healthy and happy - e.g. a plant, a seashell, a candle, a piece of fruit
- A picture of a scene that makes you feel healthy and happy -- e.g. a beach, a forest, a city you love, etc.
- A picture of a loved one, a picture of yourself that you love

These things can be anything else that might pique your interest and make you feel happy and energized. And the altar might shift as you move through your journey. Things might stay there the whole time, some items might be added, and other items might go away and never return.

Ideally, this altar will be in a place where you can look at it regularly. Some like an altar in a bathroom or on a bedside table. You might want it on a dresser in your bedroom or on your office desk. You might have something in your car if you drive a lot or you might have a small picture that you put in your wallet so you see it daily.

No matter where your altar is and what it includes, this is a place to return to. Some might sit by their altar when they meditate or when they're working on releasing stories. Others might simply light a candle on their altar for a few minutes each day, just to think about their intention before they start the busyness of life.

You may also have an altar in your house and also in your office. There's no such thing as too many altars, after all. And if you're traveling, you could always take a picture of the altar and have it on your phone or computer to look at when you need a boost.

Finding a Space for Connection

If you're not a 'thing' person, you might find a place to focus on your intention for your health and well-being. Some find it soothing to find a spot in nature where they can go and think about what they want in their life. When you can go back to the same spot again and again, you can find a grounding place that allows you to feel connected to yourself.

Allow yourself to take some time to find a spot that works for you. You may need to find a place that is away from people, or not. You might need a place that has something beautiful to look at, or not. You might need to find the right stone to sit on or the log that fits your body.

You might need to create a space for yourself in your yard or a corner of your house. This spot will be the place you return to when you need some solace or some reminder of what you're doing. You may bring things to decorate the space or you may leave small things when you visit. Sometimes called a sit spot, this place can be anywhere you like, so long as it resonates with you and feels like the right place for your needs.

Grow Outside to Grow Inside

For those who are less about sitting, you may want to seek out a way to grow things in your life instead of a place for an altar or a sit spot. You might want to plant a garden and use that time to think about your intention. You may want to focus on time with your pet to help you stay in alignment with the energy you want in your life.

You can choose to grow a plant from the seed stage to fullness or you may find that you want to take a plant that is already started to grow and keep it healthy. Or you might be a person who can take a plant that is not doing well and bring it back to health.

Get creative in the way you focus your energy. You might find you need other things to bring yourself back to the point of your process. Some people need cleaning, some need dance, some need art. What might you need? Try that. And if that doesn't work, try something else.

Getting to Know Yourself

Remember, this process of health and well-being is not just a process of the body, it's a process of better relating to yourself. The more you know and care for the body you are in, the more you will be able to support yourself well.

But really, how well do you know yourself? You might know what you like to eat or what sorts of movies you hate, but what about the deeper layers? What about the things that matter most to you? Or the things that scare you the most? When we can tap into the places that aren't normally part of conversations about health, we can get to the core of caring for our vessels.

Automatic Writing

It can help to begin with a list of questions you want to ask of yourself. Think about this process as dating yourself and finding out more about this being. You might walk into a date with some questions you ask of everyone to get to know them, so why not turn them around and ask yourself too? I might suggest skipping past the questions that talk about what you do versus who you are. So, asking yourself about your job or your hobbies is something that you can avoid. Instead, try writing out a list of questions like:

- What do you love?
- What makes you smile?
- What are you afraid of?
- What would you do if you could do anything?

And so on.

Write out a list of the questions you'd really like to know the answers to and once you have this list, get out a journal. At the top of the page, write out one question. Once that is written, start writing out the answer to the question on the paper that follows it. Don't stop writing for 5 to 10 minutes. Even if you're not sure what to say, just keep writing. You can keep repeating the question to yourself to keep yourself on track.

Write until the time is up. You don't have to go back and read it right away, but think about how the experience made you feel. Did you write things you didn't realize you'd write? Were you stumped when you didn't think you'd be stumped? What did the experience bring up for you?

- Did you notice resistance?
- Did you notice fear?
- Did you notice the small rumblings of joy and hope?
- Did you start to whisper to yourself that maybe, just maybe there are things that could happen for you?

This is a practice of letting the logical part of you fall to the side and open to the realms of expanding possibility. You can return to this practice whenever you have a question about what comes next. You can return to this practice when you're unclear or you just want more information to arrive.

Mapping Your Body

For those who are more interested in being visual, you can also utilize a practice of mapping your body. This can be done in a variety of ways, so I will offer a possibility that can be expanded to fit the container of who you are and how you are emerging in this particular moment.

You can begin with a piece of paper, of any size -- small or large. This piece of paper will contain the outline of your body as you know it today. It can be a clear representation of the way your body looks or it can be a simple outline that looks like a human body.

Within this space, begin to look at where you are present, what parts of you feel connected to who you are and what parts might have other stories to tell. You might begin with filling in the space with words or colors. Maybe some parts are brighter and some are not. If you feel called, you might fill certain parts of your drawing with images of nature because they feel they are growing and thriving. Or there might be parts of you that are less vital at the present moment. Dream into, feel into the way your body is before you. Notice what you might draw in those spaces. Only you have to know what these images mean.

Take time to get to know your body's map and the way it is rough and smooth at the same time. You might notice you have certain areas that are more present for you than others. You may notice you aren't clear on what your body feels like or what it holds right now. That's okay too. This is not a time for judging your body, its shape or its texture. This is a time to simply put into images what your body is like at the moment. I might notice that the space of my head is many colors because it's always thinking.

Or I might notice that certain parts of my body are more alive than others because of the ways I do (and don't) care for them. Allow this to be a practice and an exercise that enables you to be more present with the body you have. This beautiful body that allows you to experience the world. And while there may be moments where you believe it to be in need of more attention, you will have that time. You will make that time.

Right now, map the body as you see it, as only you know it. In that creation of an image, you will bring into perspective what needs your support and your presence.

Breath

Getting to know yourself is a study of getting to know all the things that you may not have considered previously. It's only when we slow down and make the time that we can begin to really understand who we are, outside of what others want us to be. And it can be as simple as getting to know your breath.

In guided meditations and trances I lead, the first thing I say is to be with your breath exactly as it is in that moment, without trying to fix or change it. So often, we might think we need to be a certain way or move at a certain pace. But your body is yours. Your choices are yours. Your breath is yours.

Today, your breath might be shallow and quick. Tomorrow, your breath might be slow and even. The next day, it might show up differently or move between the spaces of fast and slow. For this moment, close your eyes and notice how you breathe. Notice how your chest rises and falls. Notice if your chest moves more than your stomach with each breath, or vice versa. Allow yourself to get to know your breath as it is. In and out.

Are you more focused on the inhalation? Or the exhalation? Or both? Or neither? Allow yourself the luxury, the permission to be as you are. Let your lungs fill in the way they need to fill. And you might notice you need to breathe in more deeply to feel nourished right now. Or you might feel your breath quicken because you're paying attention more closely than usual. The breath is an automatic function of your body, feeding your blood, allowing you to have energy and life.

Allow your breath to be as it is. Try to stay focused on your breath. If you find your mind wandering into judgment or into worry, begin to count the number of inhalations you take. As your mind tries to distract you, come back to the numbers.

Your mind will wander, especially if you're not accustomed to being so present. It's okay. It's not a failure or concern. It is just the truth of the present moment. It's fine. You're fine. You're breathing and alive in the way you are right now. Continue to stay with your breath for as long as you like. Notice and accept yourself in the way you are.

Focusing on the breath (and we'll do more in later chapters) allows you to come to the present moment and back to your body. It is a way to bring your thoughts away from the past and the future. You can come into the present moment, where everything is possible. The more you come to know your breath, the more you will return to it.

Making & Keeping Promises

As we start where we are and as we start to get to know ourselves, it is helpful to build a foundation of trust. This foundation will support you as you move through your own journey. And no matter where this journey takes you, the more you can trust, the more you will grow and expand into your life.

A common piece of advice in therapeutic practices is to begin making small promises to yourself each day, promises that you keep. As you keep more promises, you will begin to trust yourself to show up for yourself. A promise can be as small as drinking a glass of water when you wake up. A promise can be as big as saying you will speak up when you have something to say. I don't know what feels big or small to you for your promises, and I trust that you will know.

It is easier to start with things you KNOW you will keep. This might be something you do every day already. You might keep these smaller promises for a few weeks before moving onto something that feels bigger for you.

I promise to write in my journal.
I promise to sit at my altar.
I promise to walk around the block once.
I promise to call or text a friend when I need help.

Find a few promises that feel doable and realistic. Starting right now, write down a promise that you will keep for yourself either today or tomorrow. At the start of the day, you can remind yourself of the promise and then check back in with yourself toward the end of the day to see if you kept it.

And if you don't keep your promise one day, notice why you didn't do it. At first, you may notice you have resistance that sounds like 'that's silly' or 'that isn't going to help.' Again, this is normal, even expected when you're not used to trusting yourself or you've been told you can't trust yourself. But do it anyway. Take the time to show up for yourself. Take the time to be reliable and consistent for yourself. Not only does this help you trust yourself, but it also helps you remember that even when things aren't going the way you want them to go, you can rely on yourself. You have your own back. Even if you step into a difficult place, you will show up for you.

* * *

You are starting a grand journey and the starting place can be very exciting. It is also the place where you might feel vulnerable and nervous. If you're like so many others, you may have tried to show up for yourself before, only to feel let down. And if this sounds like you, take a breath, come back to the present moment, and know that you can make a different choice today. You can choose you.

Your Body as the Foundation

Take a moment to become aware of your hand. You might look at it. You might trace the skin with the other hand's fingers. You might feel the sunlight or the wind or the way it rests on a chair. Your hand is a part of your beautiful and wondrous body. Even if you feel your body is not where you want it to be or it has limits you wish it didn't have, your body is the vessel of your wonder. Your body is the container of your being in this world right now.

Your body is the place that is your home. It is the collection of chemical processes that happen like magic, all to support your life. There are mysteries that doctors and scientists haven't solved. The body is a place that shifts and changes over the years, sometimes without clear reasons and sometimes with habit and action. We look to the body to help us in our unfolding and in our beginning.

What I want to make clear before we begin is that there is no ideal way for the body to look or to feel. I can't tell you what's right for you or what's best for you. All I can say is that your body is impacted by the choices you make -- and when you want to prepare for a complete revitalization of your being, your physical health is essential. Your body needs to be strong to hold the work you are doing.

Making Strong the Vessel

Once upon a time in my spiritual training, I was told a story of a tradition I am a part of and one that I am still studying today (and likely will do for the rest of my life). I remember talking about the practices of this tradition and how it moved my body in new ways. I'd also heard that this practice often caused people to lose themselves.

I saw this show up as people losing their sense of self or as losing their sense of groundedness. They would say things that were out of integrity with their practice or they would simply be mean because they felt like doing so. When I talked to another student about this, they offered that some people's vessels aren't strong enough to hold the energy of that work. While there are nuances to this statement and certainly there could be a longer conversation about differing abilities, what I took from this is the idea that the body needs to be prepared as much as the mind or heart.

If a person is not doing the work of caring for themselves, their body may not be as strong as they would like it to be. And as such, the body then does not offer the foundation of support when things are challenging. I've seen this in the work that is done with trauma in the body. When a person experiences trauma, one of the common pieces of advice is to take care of the physical body. Eat well, move more, and get enough sleep.

Trauma is an exhausting experience, and so is the everyday experience of life's challenges. It can be harder to navigate rough spots when the body isn't fortified. During these periods of stress, the body's immune system can be depleted, you can get sick, and you can have challenges maintaining calm.

To be clear, being in trauma and being in life are hard enough without hearing that you should be doing more. I get that. Beyond the stories of judgment, you might begin to feel right now is the offering of coming into a better relationship with your body.

Coming into a relationship that looks like taking care of yourself as much as you take care of others. Think about the last time you saw a friend struggling. While you may not have told them what to do, you may have thought about how they could care for themselves. In hard times, the very least/most we can offer to ourselves is care and attention.

We can seek out nourishing foods. We can make sure to move our bodies in a way that feels supportive. We can make sure to rest. None of this removes the stress or the worry, but a healthy body is one that will not react as harshly. It will be able to support us as we move through the things we need to move through at the moment.

Why the Body Needs Your Strength

Just as it is wise to keep small promises to yourself to build trust with yourself, showing up for the physical needs of your body will allow you to believe in your ability to support yourself. A body that is strong is a body that can hold not only energy and power, but also faith in the unknown.

A body that is strong and nourished is a body that can bounce back from things that happen -- expected and unexpected. A body that is strengthened by your choices is a body that will be able to move ahead confidently. And while there will always be times when you feel out of sorts or when you feel you are lost in your life; a healthy and strong body will help you get to the next place -- even if you're not quite sure where that is yet.

A strong body is one that will also be adaptable as you will need to shift things in your life. Relationships have troubles, work lives can be difficult, and death happens. While those are often moments when we focus outward and away from the bodies we have, if we are already taking care of ourselves, we can more easily stay on track.

Think of this support of your body as not something that takes away from other things as they happen, but rather these supportive actions will allow you to take on more. (Of course, you're not going to be able to take on EVERYTHING that happens. But we'll get to that later.)

It's also clear how wellness is linked to the way you take care of your body. Though it's true you will not be able to avoid sickness or low energy days, the more you can take care of your body on days when you already feel well, the more likely you are to have more days when you feel healthy. Some studies have also shown that the more proactive you are in taking care of your body, the more you will be able to avoid illness and fatigue. This does not mean it's easy to prioritize your body every day. But it is worth it. You are worth it.

Like the little promises you want to make to yourself every day, your body needs you to stand up for it. To listen and to respond to what it really needs. And if you don't know what your body needs, now is the time to learn how to get quiet enough to know what's best. You can start by simply taking note of what your body tells you every day. If this is not something that you've done before, no worries. You can easily pick up this practice by setting aside 5 minutes a day to listen to your body. Just close your eyes and let your mind relax. When you do, try to push aside the thoughts that tell you that you 'should' or 'should not' do something.

This is not about what you've read on the news or seen on the Internet as the next greatest tip for your well-being. Instead, you need to think about the unique needs of your body. And your body will tell you.

Close your eyes and allow your breath to be what it needs to be for the time you will spend listening to your body. Scan your body to notice where it is tense, where it hurts, and where it is hungry. When you notice something, take a moment to try to describe it without trying to make meaning of it. For example, if you notice your knee is tense, you might describe the quality of it. *Oh, there's pain here and some tension around the kneecap. There's a slight pinch in the area behind my knee.* Allow the sensation to be as it is. It's very easy to start to talk with your body about how it hurts because you failed in some way. Or because you're a certain age. Or because you didn't ------.

It's no wonder we have troubles listening to our bodies. If you were talking to someone and all they did was criticize what you said, you might stay away from them in the future too.

When you do notice judgmental thoughts creep in, just let

them fall away. Let them be thoughts that exist and also thoughts that can be released just as easily as they come in.

It will take practice. It will take time for your body to trust that you are listening. But keep showing up.

As you sit there and you listen, you can focus on all of the areas that are giving you information or you might focus on one area at a time. That's up to you. It can help to ask that area of your body questions once you have identified something to notice:

- What do you need?
- What are you missing?
- What can I do to help?

Just as you might ask a friend what they need when they're feeling under the weather, talk to your body in the same way. Once you've asked the questions, listen. You may need to wait for a while to hear anything, but you will. You might learn that your knee wants to move more. Or that your hips are out of alignment, which is impacting your knee. Even the smallest bit of information is important, so listen to it all and allow it to be welcome.

It can help to write things down after you've listened. And it is also wise to thank your body for the information. Thank it for the ways in which it holds knowledge and promise you will do your best to listen in the future. Like any practice, the more you do this, the better you will get at it. Soon, you will be able to listen to your body in real time, rather than having to set aside time to 'chat.'

I also encourage you to spend time listening to your body as you 'hear' it during the day. Notice where your energy grows and where it wanes. Listen to the way your body follows the energy of the day and the obstacles it faces. Notice the way it responds and notice the way you listen to what it really needs.

This is a practice of showing up for yourself -- and when you show up for your body, it becomes easier to show up during more difficult or confusing times too. After all, when the world is confusing and unclear, you can come back to your body. You can come back to the present moment and ask what your body needs. That foundation it provides is the beginning of a partnership -- one that supports growth and self-discovery and joy.

How to Hold the Energy of Your Life

Instead of looking at the world as points on a schedule or tasks on a To Do list, we can begin to look at life as the movement of energy. Some days, we start with a large container of energy and other days, we might only get a teaspoon. In a world that wants us to do more, be more, and produce more, it becomes commonplace to find ways to take the smallest amount of energy and make it last all day. While this is common, it does not mean it's healthy.

Another way to approach your life is to get to know the energy you have and the energy it takes for you to approach different activities. Some of us are energized by phone calls, for example, while others might be wiped out by them.

By learning to track the energy it takes for you to do what you need to do, you can hold onto more energy and move with the way your body already likes to move. But this can sound nebulous when you've thought about crossing things off as a measure of a life well-managed. Let's try something new.

When you want to get to know something better, you need to examine it, watch it, and figure out how it works. The best way to do this with your body is to start by tracking what your energy does. You can do this by writing out what you do every day for a certain period of time. You might choose to do this for a few days or a week or longer.

It can help to get a journal that you can write your everyday activities in, but then assign them a color or symbol of how much energy they take out of you. You might start with this system first and then adapt in a way that makes more sense to you.

Red / yellow / green ... Write out your schedule and assign each task a color based on the energy you think it will take. This might mean that red items are those that are energy-depleting while green are those that are energy-restoring. But don't stop there, at the end of the day, add in the color that was actually right for how the day went. For example, the meeting that you thought was going to be energizing may have been depleting. Note what you experience before and after to get a sense of the energetic pattern of your life.

After you have tracked things for a few days, notice if there are patterns in how your days ended up happening. You may notice that your days are redder in the afternoon and then there are green spots in the evening.

What you're doing with this exercise is to find out when your natural energy movements are and how they shift over the course of your choices and the days of the week. It's common to have a lot of energy in the morning and then less in the evening. Or you might be the opposite.

When you have a clearer idea of your energy movements, you can begin to schedule things to follow these patterns. If you're more in tune with your natural patterns, you are less likely to feel out of sync with your life. You will be able to get into the flow of your life more easily and you will end days feeling accomplished, versus exhausted. (Now, this is not to say that the goal of this practice is to increase your productivity. The goal of this practice is to support the natural needs of your body. You *may* find that in supporting your body, you can also get more done.)

As you begin to see the patterns of your life, you can begin to schedule things in a way that supports your energetic flow. You might notice too that certain things will always take energy away from you. When this is the case, you might decide to only schedule those things once a week -- or you could delegate those items to someone else.

You might decide that you need to do high-brain power things in the morning and less brain-intensive things in the afternoon. You might decide you need to write and create in the middle of the night because that works for you. You may notice you need to do something completely different. No matter what you decide you need, the more you can pay attention and respond to your body, the more it will support your needs in return.

Other ideas for tracking your energy is to list out all of the things you have to do on a regular basis. You may want to rank them in terms of the joy they bring you, knowing full well that not everything is a joyful practice to everyone.

Once you have this ranking on a piece of paper, you might decide to prioritize the joyful items in your life. You might decide that you need to do at least one of these each day. Or you if you have a day that looks to be 'joyless,' you might make it important that the rest of the day includes things that make you smile. This is not so much about balance as it is about supporting what your body and mind already love. When you do that, you will not only feel better, but you will also trust that when things are hard that you will make time for things that are beautiful too.

Manifesting Your Dreams

The strong vessel is one that is ready to hold large and amazing things. What those things look like to you is unique and individual. There are no goals that you 'should' be looking at outside of what makes you feel fulfilled and happy in your life. But it's hard to not be impacted by the greater world and what it seems to think we need. And it's hard to not compare ourselves to the way others act around us. Plus, it's hard to see someone else's happiness and think that we need to do what they did in order to secure our own joy.

But this isn't about anyone else but you. Though you might begin with chasing someone else's dream, I encourage you to find your own. I challenge and even dare you to consider what makes you truly happy. What are your dreams? And more importantly, what are your dreams right now? Not tomorrow and not next year. In this precious moment, what are your dreams?

Dreams and goals will change. They will shift and sometimes it will feel as though we have outgrown them. Of course, we are always changing and that means what we want will change. Or it might just look different. Or it might deepen and expand.

But how do we shut out the dreams of others and the expectations of others? How do we call into ourselves the truth of our dreams? How do we call into our hearts the things we only whisper to ourselves?

Perhaps surprisingly, we don't begin with creating a list of our dreams. We start with getting quiet. We start with shutting out the influences we know and the influences we don't know. We start by backing away from others and backing away from expectations. Getting quiet begins with letting go of expectations. One way to do this is to write down all of the things you were told growing up you had to be:

- I have to have a steady career.
- I have to make a certain amount of money.
- I have to be debt free.
- I have to own a house.
- I have to have children.

Write down all of the things you were told you needed to do or to have. Write down all of the things you weren't told you had to have, but you learned you 'needed' to have through friends, colleagues, and the media. Let it all go onto a piece of paper. Or draw them. Or get some clay and make a shape that represents them -- it doesn't really matter how you do it. Find a way to collect them so you can see just how many expectations have been placed upon you. When you see this, it can become clear why you have trouble naming your dreams -- the ones that are only for you.

It's loud in the land of expectation. It's noisy in the land of should-do and why-aren't-you-doing-this. And because we are people who want to make others happy, we want to listen to others and consider their advice. Even when it's bad advice. Even when the advice is just bad advice, they got from someone else. So, let's drop that advice. Let's get back to us. To the vessel that already knows things and knows (at least for now) what it wants.

Dreaming big is scary. When we dream big, we begin to feel all the feelings. We might start to think about the ways we could screw it up and the ways we might be asking for too much. But asking for what you want is not asking for too much. It is asking for your life to be the way you want it to be, for the way you deserve it to be. And while there is always the chance that you won't get EVERYTHING you want, asking for what is true for you allows you to bring dreams closer and closer.

Calling in What You Want

The asking can be the hardest part after admitting you have dreams in the first place. Sure, it might be great to have things you want, but if you start to ask for them, that means there is a chance you won't get them. And for many the idea that they might try for what they want and not get it sounds more painful. After all, to get close to joy and not get it feels ouchy.

I want to tell you I understand. I do. I know what it means to stop and say I'm worth the joy I want for others. I know what it means to ask for big things and to immediately regret calling that into the universe. I know what it means to not want to be let down. Again. Or again. But...bravery has its own rewards. What we don't ask for will never come to be.

Even if this practice of calling in what you want seems a little strange, I invite you to try it anyway. Even if you feel uncomfortable and doubtful, I want you to try and follow the motions anyway. Just because you don't believe in yourself right now doesn't mean the universe doesn't believe in you. I believe the universe knows you are human and knows you are going to have doubts. I know the universe can 'see' past the trembling in your voice and begin to open the way to your dreams. So, show up and see what arrives for you. Show up with your fear, with your doubt, and with your worry. Show up as you are.

Calling in what you want starts with choosing something to call into your life. Many people get stuck here because they don't want to choose the 'wrong' thing. It doesn't matter. Choose something. Choose a dream that has been calling your name since you were young. Or choose a dream that just arrived in your consciousness as something you'd really like. Choose something.

Once you choose something, describe it in detail. Take time to create a visceral experience of it. In the Hawaiian Huna tradition, there is a practice of visualization that allows this to happen. Engage all of your senses in the scene of your dream. Take time to see it in your mind. Take time to hear what can be heard. Take time to feel and touch what you can. Taste it. Smell it. Take all of your senses to the dream you have.

Allow the dream to become as vivid as reality, and so vivid that it is hard to determine if it's just a dream or something that's already real. Come back to this scene, filling it in with new details and new sensations. Come back to this scene, ideally before bed so it can get into your brain and your nighttime dreaming. Fall asleep to the description you have created.

With each moment you spend in this dream, you will call the dream forward. You will call it into existence. You will begin to notice things happening that remind you of what you want or you might notice things happen that bring you closer to your dream. Others notice they are able to feel the dream within reach. And others might notice they are able to believe in their dreams more easily. All of these things are good. All of these experiences are helpful. All of these things are confidence boosting, not just for you, but also for your dreams. I like to think of dreams as energy and when you send energy to your dreams, they will send energy back to you.

You might want to feed your dreams in some way, feed them with attention and with faith. You might continue to think about what the dream might look like, how it might arrive in your life and how it might impact other parts of your life.

Much like the idea of breathing life into something, the intention and attention you give to your dreams is the energy of creation. This is the energy of calling in what you really want, and calling it in so loudly that it begins to call back to you.

Nourishment

Your body is the foundation of your existence and what helps to carry you from one moment to the other. It is powerful, it has needs, and it requires your attention as much as your dreams do. And it requires nourishment. Fuel for power.

And here's where it gets tricky. There is no one way, no right way to eat -- no matter what you've been told. There is no magical way to nourish yourself so you can get everything you want. But your body does need you to nourish it. Like we've already talked about, it's not about following a certain method and it's not about listening to everyone else. In fact, trying to keep up with all of the advice about eating is confusing at best -- infuriating, at worst.

Instead, let's look for a new way. Let's look for a customized way to support the way you feel in each day. Just as we have in so many other areas (and we will continue to do), we need to figure out what we already know -- and we need to listen.

If you're a person who likes to eat on the run or someone who doesn't have a lot of time to eat, you might not give your food too much thought. You might think of it as something to keep you going and the easier it is to chew or grab, the better. There's nothing inherently wrong with this, so long as you feel good in the end. I am not going to tell you to eat a certain way or to avoid certain foods. I can tell you what works for me, but even that is not advice I would want from someone else.

Instead, let's talk about what foods feel good to your body -- your unique body. To find out, it helps to keep a food diary. Ignore the calories and other information (unless that brings you happiness) and focus instead of what the food feels like in your body before and after you eat it:

- Do you look forward to eating it?
- Do you feel a duty to eat it?
- How do you feel after eating this food?
- How do you feel hours after eating this food?

The more you can look at what you eat, the more you will be able to decide what is most nourishing to your particular body. For example, I know that quinoa is good for me. I know it has protein in it and it is a great way to fuel a body. But it doesn't work for my body. It makes me feel bloated and icky. Since I know this, I avoid it. I am not allergic to it. I like the taste and texture, but it does not work for me.

After so much time eating it anyway because it was so popular and revered, I finally said to myself -- why? Why am I eating something I do not like and that does not (apparently) like me? So, I stopped eating it. And my body was very happy that I made that choice. On some level, my body realized that I listened to it and it was more willing to give me information about other foods. Like any relationship, building trust requires listening and acting on that information.

What to Eat

When you start to track your food to see how your body responds, you can create a list of things that feel good and don't feel good. Like the Red, Yellow, Green system for tracking your energy, you can use those colors for your eating. Perhaps Red is what doesn't feel good and Green is what does, while Yellow is a food that is somewhere in the middle.

And I would also invite you to think about the source of your food. Though processed foods might make you feel good, and you are well within your right to eat them as you like, those foods may not help your body in the long run. And I know you may not be in a place where it is easy to access fresh food all the time. Or you might have a budget or not have the time to cook.

With this in mind, I'm still not going to tell you what to do. What I am going to offer is that it can be wise to consider the nutritional value of the foods you take into your body. You might want to look at the vitamins and minerals. You might want to look at the sugar content or the fiber. See what your foods include and then decide if those are things that are important to you.

You might decide you want to have more vitamins and minerals in your diet, so focus on foods that offer this. Check to see how they make you feel and then continue to eat them if you like the way they worked for you. It can start with a simple curiosity about your current energy levels. When do you feel your best? What did you eat that day? When do you feel awful? Do you notice a connection with the foods you ate that day or that week? Get curious and learn what your body already tells you. You might find it's been asking you for a vegetable or a piece of fruit. Or maybe it just wants a cupcake every now and then. Your body knows.

How to Eat

No matter how you decide to eat and what you decide to eat, it helps to become more present when you do eat. So many of us are disconnected when we finally find the time to nourish our bodies. We're looking at our phones, our computers, the TV, or some other outside information source. Because of this, we don't necessarily experience the food we eat. We might taste a few bites, but the rest simply happen -- outside of our awareness. This causes us to be less skilled at hearing our body's cues for flavor and fullness. We need to get present and eat more consciously. This might require changes in the way we act during mealtimes. Here are some things you may want to choose to help you become more present.

- Get away from the technology when you eat - When you can walk away from your phone, computer, TV, etc. you can bring yourself fully present to the experience of eating. You can become part of the process and taste everything that the food has to offer. It is also common to slow down when you eat in this present state.
- Before you eat - Stop and take a moment to look at what you are eating. What do you notice? What surprises you? Or you may want to stop and consider the scents that arise from the meal before you. What do you smell? What does steam feel like from hot food? Can you experience the coolness of cold or chilled food?
- Become mindful as you eat - As you settle your mind and stop the distractions, you may want to turn eating into a mindfulness practice. You can do this by thinking about each bite as an opportunity to learn something about the food. What does it taste like? What is the texture? What is the temperature? How does it feel in the mouth?
- Take smaller bites - You can also become more aware of your eating when you take smaller bites and slow down the process. Food is supposed to be enjoyable and the more time you can offer to the experience, the more you

will taste and feel with each bite.

- Eat alone - When you are first starting to eat more mindfully, it can help to eat on your own. Find a place where you can eat regularly and come back to that place, as though eating were a ritual.

You might also notice that eating in the same place will help you become more aware of the experience. And it is ideal to not eat at your desk or a place that isn't specifically for food -- whenever possible. The more you bring your awareness to eating, the more you will be able to create a connection between nourishment and pleasure. The more you can bring yourself to the action of giving your body what it needs, the more you will want to find ways to better nourish all of your cells.

Weight is not a Measure of your Health or Worth

Because this is a story many of us know, I want to bring up the conversation of weight. As you may have noticed, I don't talk about weight. I don't equate certain weights with health and I don't condone weight loss to achieve some certain goal set by society or an outdated chart.

Weight is just a number. Just a number. Though the world might continue to tell you and so many of us that our weight needs to be a certain number in order to be 'good,' this is not true. You can be X weight and run marathons. You can be X weight and have nutritional deficiencies. It's just a number.

Some people's weight is influenced by metabolism or by autoimmune conditions. Some people have trouble eating because of medications or illnesses or life issues. Some people have swelling because of medications or illnesses or injuries. What you see on the outside is not a measure of value or wellness inside. If you find you have trouble separating weight from health, I invite you to stop weighing yourself. Really. Stop weighing yourself and focus more on what your body tells you.

If it is happy and you are well, then you are the right weight.

The size of your clothing doesn't matter, unless it matters to you. If you want to do something for yourself, do it. But if you're doing it because of someone else or because you feel you HAVE to, then I gently encourage you to consider coming back to what's right for you.

It might sound as though I'm minimizing this conversation. It's not easy to just stop worrying about what others or society thinks. It takes time to dismantle the structures and the ideas that we have been told for years, perhaps for our entire lives. It's hard to disconnect from the images we see in the media. It's easy to say the number doesn't matter...and harder to remember this when we're not happy with a number we see for ourselves. The messages we have been given are deeply carved into our consciousness. This is another reason for spending time focusing on how food makes you feel versus what it does to your shape. When you can focus on the experience that is true for you, it will get easier to ignore the weight question. And it can also help to surround yourself with people with similar interests and goals.

Consistency & Listening to Your Body

Nourishing your body well might be something that comes naturally to you. You might already know what to eat and what feels good for you. It might be a question now of how to be consistent. For those who feel they need more help or support with eating well, you might need to spend more time listening and tracking. You might need to try different foods than you have been eating. You may need to completely rearrange what your nourishment plan has looked like for years.

This might be a place where you need to focus before you can go any further. This is fine. I encourage you to do what feels best for you. Coming into a better or more intentional relationship with your body is a step that can't be rushed or skipped. It's a step that needs care and attention. If you take your time in caring for yourself and getting to know your body's needs, you will find the rest of the work much easier. So much of this health and well-being journey is about listening to our inner knowing. Take your time. You are learning about the home of yourself. You can take the time you need.

Movement

The body is designed to move with its joints, its muscles, and its electrical impulses of messaging. While some bodies have different ways of moving and being in the world, the research shows that bodies that are active in some way are bodies that are healthy. (Let's say too, that bodies that can't move easily or at all are still able to be active. However, as these are states of being of which I am not as familiar and I am not a medical professional, I will need to suggest talking to professionals who are trained in these areas.)

There is a physics rule which states that an object at rest will stay at rest, while an object in motion will stay in motion unless an equal or opposing force acts upon it. We could move this phrase into the activity of a body and state that a body that moves more often is a body that will continue to be active.

Stop and think about how much you move your body right now. Are you moving it when you need to do something or are you trying to find ways to stay as still as possible? Are you seeking out opportunities to get outside and to engage your muscles? Bodies that are able to move and that do take time to move are bodies that stay flexible and strong. And bodies that are flexible and strong support the mind and the heart of the human. As our breath supports our being, our muscles and bones support our movement. When we take the time to engage them and to use them, we create alignment with the power of our intention.

Knowing Your Body's Needs

Like anything we do for ourselves, we need to think about what our body needs to be happy and healthy. We might find that we need a long walk once a week to feel vital or we might need to run six miles a day. What you do is up to you and up to the needs of your body. And like anything else, it's not about trying to achieve some certain measure of fitness or strength. If you want to be able to run a marathon, that's great. If you want to be able to move around with your children or friends without running out of breath, that's great. If you just want to be able to sit on the floor for an hour without getting stiff, that's a great goal too -- when it feels good to you.

Let's begin with a clear conversation about what your body needs to feel good. Again, it can help to check in with your body over the course of a week to see what makes it feel good and what makes it feel not-so-good:

- Do you feel better when you have exercised during the day?
- How much movement feels good?
- How much do you sit during the day?

While fitness trackers are not accessible to everyone, they measure things you may want to track too. You might want to check to see how many hours you spend without getting up. For those with desk jobs, tracking this might give you some information you already know or information you hadn't realized. Most trackers will compile information on steps, movement, exercise, and heart rate. You can also check these things on your own or with the help of phone applications -- if you have the ability and the desire. Or you can simply track the minutes you spend moving around during a day. Estimation is fine. There are no grades for this work after all. The only person who might be assessing you is...you.

The scientific research around sitting for long periods seems to be moving toward the idea that we should be moving around as much as we can. But let's emphasize that -- as much as we can. Not everyone is able to get up every hour due to the needs of their work or due to the way their body works. What is clear is that activity of some sort for a period of time that feels good for you is wise. When you can take the time to track what your body might need and what your body might want, you can begin to bring this information into your life more.

You might notice on days when you are stressed, you need more movement. Or when you haven't slept, you need to get outside once in a while. Or you might see that days when you are busy, you may need to move more, but you also need time to rest earlier. You may notice that certain activities are more invigorating than others. You may see that some activities are better at different times of the day.

While you may be bored of tracking yourself and watching yourself, there is so much information to help inspire what you might need to do or what you might want to do next for yourself. The more you know, the more you can do.

Knowing Your Body's Limits

Your body is your unique body. While there are books upon books and magazines and websites and social media pages, etc. that will tell you how to support your body, you are the best expert. You know what your body feels like, how it responds to movement, and how it has acted in the past. This is not to say that you can't change where you're at right now if you want to, but you are the best judge of what the best first step might be.

Think back to a time when you felt healthy and well. (If you can't think of one, we'll figure out a plan in a moment, no matter where you're beginning.) Think about what you did, what it felt like, and how you managed to stay on track with the activities you did. When you think about this time, what feelings does it bring up? What does it make you want to do right now? Are you eager to try that sort of plan again? Are you more interested in how you felt versus what you did? You might journal on these questions or you might simply think about them as you consider what your body might need from you.

For those who don't have a template for wellness, we're going to start from the ground up. First things first, before you attempt any sort of change in your diet or exercise, it's best to talk to a doctor -- especially if you have health conditions or you've had troubles with new programs in the past. Get checked out -- and from there, you can move forward.

For some people, it can help to think about physical activity in three different parts:

- Movement
- Strength
- Flexibility

While some might call movement 'cardio,' I feel it's better to expand that activity a bit since not everyone is excited by the idea of making their heart beat faster than they'd like. Movement is where you move your body in the space it is in. This could look like walking, running, swimming, biking, or dancing. It could look like other activities that you enjoy, so long as you are moving your body in some way.

As you do this, you will need to engage your breath a bit more and your heart is likely to beat faster. This is due to your body needing more fuel and more oxygen to keep going. The heart pumps harder to get oxygen to your cells and muscles, while your lungs take in more air to keep the supply of oxygen to where it needs to be. All of this is normal. Of course, if you feel uncomfortable or you feel pain, stop what you're doing and check in with your doctor.

Most fitness magazines will tell you to exercise for at least

30 minutes, 3 times a week. And other professionals will advise you to move your body every day. What works for you? What feels good for you? What can you put into your schedule as a gift back to your body? What can you do that feels sustainable and energizing versus challenging?

You might start with just 5 minutes of movement a day until that becomes 10 minutes or more. You may find you need to exercise every other day or just on the weekends. Whatever works for you is great when it feels good to you.

It can help to add in some strength exercises to power up your muscles. You don't need to spend time in a gym to do this (or you could). You can do things as simple as standing in front of a chair and pretending to sit down, but then come up as soon as your bottom hits the chair. And you can do some pushups on your knees instead of your toes (or even against the wall). These two exercises alone will work your leg muscles and your upper body muscles. Not too bad and not too time consuming. And if these don't appeal to you, just doing things like lifting groceries will help your muscles. Lifting things that are heavy, but not overly heavy, will engage your muscles and build your strength.

The final piece to activity is flexibility. So often, people call this stretching -- and that is certainly true. But you can also do things like yoga or Pilates or simply reaching for your toes once a day. In cultivating flexibility, you simply need to extend your muscles more and release any stiffness you might have.

Listen to your body to see what it needs, where it is stiff, and where it might need some extra stretch. Think about the way that this stretching helps you elongate your body -- and also your mind. In all of this, the body might be moving, but the brain is following. You are moving energy and that means you are shifting the way you think and the way you interact in the world.

It bears repeating to say there are no rules to movement -- only that you should do what feels good for you. If you have been feeling stuck in your life, perhaps moving your physical body can clear away the stiffness of your energetic life. If you have been feeling like you don't know where to go, maybe going for a walk will help you find the way.

Movement as a Practice

While there are no perfect plans and no schedules that will make your body work perfectly, I invite the possibility that you can add some sort of movement to every day. I offer the permission to move your body in the space it's in for some time each and every day. When you come back to your body, when you show up for your body, you show that it can trust you and it can show up for you too. So often, the body becomes a vehicle for doing things, versus something that needs to be tended to.

We can get so caught up in criticizing our bodies when they don't do what they are supposed to do, while also doing things that our bodies don't like. Perhaps we can think about taking care of our bodies just as we might take care of any relationship:

- What do you need?
- What do I need?
- How can I help?
- Is this still working?
- Is there something else we can try?

Sinking into the questions of your body's needs and its wishes from you will allow you to find the ways in which you can offer responses. You can offer the possibility that the relationship can be mended, the relationship can be deepened, and the relationship can become collaborative. Showing up takes work and it takes presence. Your body has done this for you. And you can return the favor(s).

Hydration

It seems to be common knowledge that our bodies are made up of mostly water, and because of this, we have been told it is important to drink enough water each day. While this is a consistent message, it is not something that many people listen to or apply.

The advice to drink water is something that seems so common and as such, I cringe to offer it. But even in my spiritual training, it is a piece of advice that shows up as a way to restore energy, to clear energy, and to bring myself into balance:

- If I am not hydrated, I cannot think clearly.
- If I am not hydrated, I cannot digest food properly.
- If I am not hydrated, I cannot have the energy I need or expect.

Drinking water is a part of my spiritual practice every morning -- though it's not a lot of water. I do a practice in which I put anxieties or worries into the water and ask a deity to transform them into energy I can use. And then I drink the water, which has been transformed, and I allow that to rest in my body as fuel instead of discomfort or worry.

The amount of water we should be drinking is hotly debated. There was one point in time where the advice of 8 glasses of water a day was the standard. But as people began to question this piece of advice, no one could find scientific proof for it. So, the advice is a little inconsistent. I might offer that choosing the amount of water to drink is based on what you feel you need... but also that you need more water than you think you do:

- Do you live in a dry area?
- Do you move around a lot?
- Do you sweat a lot during the day?
- Do you find you're tired often?

- Do you find you have trouble digesting the food you've eaten?
- Do you have muscle pain or use chiropractic services often?

All of these things might require your body to use more water than the traditional advised amount. So, you may want to try drinking the 'accepted' 8 glasses of water a day and see how that changes the way you feel. If it feels better, stick with that. If you still feel thirsty, try drinking more. While there is some risk of drinking too much water and upsetting your electrolytes, if you are eating regularly and not drinking gallons at a time, it is very unlikely you would wander into drinking too much water.

If you're a person who doesn't like to drink water because it's too cold, too tasteless, and too boring, here are some tips:

- Drink water at room temperature by sitting out a bottle overnight to drink in the morning.
- Add lemon, lime, cucumber, or mint to each cup of water.
- Make a game of it by challenging a partner or friend to a certain number of glasses a day.
- Add one glass of water a day until you reach the amount that's right for you.
- Find a pretty glass or bottle to use.
- Add ice if you like things cold.
- Try filtering your water with a pitcher filter.

And notice how this change in caring for your body helps you. You may notice more energy and less inflammation overall. You might notice you can sleep more easily or that you have fewer digestive troubles. You might also notice you can think more clearly and your muscles aren't as sore or stiff.

Water is a lubricator and an essential part of our being. And while there is water in coffee, tea, milk, and other beverages, you may want to stick with just water to make sure you're getting enough hydration every day. Things with caffeine, for example, have a slight dehydrating effect.

It can help to adjust your water intake based on the activities you are doing each day. For example, if you are more or less active, adjust your water. If the humidity is higher or lower, adjust your intake. Try to create a responsive action to this habit and you will find your body much happier.

Sleep

While sleep is so precious and so fleeting for many of us, it is also a place where we can try to outsmart our body's natural rhythms. Whether we try to address a lack of sleep with more caffeine or sugar, or we try to sleep longer on certain days to 'make up' sleep, one thing is clear -- if we don't sleep enough and regularly, our bodies will let us know.

Sleep is essential for resetting our brains, for repairing our bodies, and for helping us return to balance. When we lose out on sleep, it can decrease our mental function, our immune function, and our energy levels. You already know what it feels like to miss out on sleep. You know how your body responds and how you try to answer that response. Often, we try to push through. But our bodies will find ways to stop us from doing so.

Like other ways we come into relationship with our bodies, we need to figure out what works best for us -- and what our bodies have (often) been screaming at us to do. Let's start with the question of how much sleep we need to get. It depends. All of our bodies are wired differently based on genetics. And many of us can't sleep the often-recommended number of hours due to our life circumstances or choices.

The most common piece of advice for sleep is to get 7 to 8 hours for adults. Those who are 'older' adults, whatever that means, may be able to get less sleep and younger humans need more sleep to continue to grow and develop. But even in this series of recommendations, it is confusing to know what's ideal. Some people are able to get little sleep and feel great, while others need a lot of sleep to feel functional. The question becomes: what works for you?

Like so much of this physical caretaking of ourselves, we can likely look to our body for the answers we seek. We can think back to when we feel good in the morning and how much sleep that required. We can think about the times when we felt awful and we can remember the hours of sleep we didn't get.

Stop and think about the hours of sleep that make you feel at your best. It may have changed since you were younger or it may have changed with different activities or schedules you have. Along with all of the tracking of food and movement, you can also track the hours of sleep you get each night to see how that feels in the morning. It can be very helpful to wake up, write down the hours of sleep you got, and then write down how refreshed you feel after an hour of being awake. (So many of us will still feel tired upon waking, but will get more energized as we move our bodies, so tracking how we feel after truly waking up can help provide a more accurate picture.)

Over the course of a month, see how much you sleep and how many days you feel good about this number. You might find you aren't getting the sleep you really need. You may notice you're spending much of your time getting more tea or coffee in order to make it through a day. But things can change.

Not getting enough sleep can be traced to a few things:

- Poor sleep hygiene
- Stress and anxiety
- Not following your body's energy rhythm

Let's face it, we often think we should be able to sleep as soon as we go to bed. And when we can't do that, we will pull out a phone or tablet or computer to help us get sleepy. But what we're coming to realize is that the brightness of the screen is disrupting our ability to send a signal to our body that it's sleep time. The bright lights make our bodies think it's still light out and thus that we should be awake. And this is where the advice that many people ignore begins.

We need to stop the pattern of confusing our bodies with too much light. We can do this by creating a very dark and quiet space in our bedroom. This requires turning off any electronics at least an hour before bed. To be even more helpful, you can move any electronics out of the bedroom to stop you from being tempted to peek when you can't sleep right away. When you do this, your body will begin to slow down and know it's time to sleep soon.

In an ideal world, you would have a consistent bedtime that will also help with your sleep hygiene. When you change the time you go to bed, it can cause your body to become confused about the cycle of the day. When you have a consistent bedtime, you will be able to shift from awake to sleepy more easily.

You will also want to have a bed that is comfortable and cool. When it is too warm in a bedroom, the body can feel as though it should still be awake. When the body is cooler, it becomes calmer and you breathe more deeply, as in sleep. Try to keep the bedroom slightly cooler and perhaps have only enough blankets to be comfortable, but not warm.

Some find it helpful to have a shower or bath before bed to instigate a cooler core temperature. When the outside of the body is warmed by hot water, the body tries to cool things down, which can activate sleepiness because the core tries to get cooler.

As part of the going to sleep ritual, you can also have something you do every night before bed. This could mean listening to soothing music, meditating, using some aromatherapy spray or a diffuser, or reading. You might do this activity for a certain period of time and then shut off the lights at a certain time. And just because you have a sleep routine or ritual doesn't mean it will always work. When you're first introducing this sort of practice, it can take a while for your body to respond. But it's worth the effort, so be patient. You will be rewarded with deeper, more restorative sleep.

But even with all of the best sleep hygiene practices, if you come to bed with worry and anxiety, you are likely to have trouble sleeping. You might have a mind that wants to focus on everything but the act of slowing down. While there may be no way to solve all of the problems of the world before you go to bed, you can find a way to put them to rest so you can sleep.

- Worry box / notepad
- Affirmation / quote
- Ritual of removal

One of the easiest ways to get rid of worries is to give them a place where they will not be forgotten. Often, our brains will continue to ruminate on things because we don't have an end point. Or we're concerned that without a solution, we will never come back to the problem. Before you go to bed, write out all of the things you're worried about and put them in a box or a journal you can close. You can even put this box or notebook in another room away from you. Allow them to be where they can be returned to, but where they will not continue to upset you.

You can also find a quote or an affirmation that will allow you to move the worrisome thoughts out of your mind. Things like 'I am calm' and 'I am ready to rest' or similar thoughts can help you slow down the mind that wants to focus on other things. Remind yourself that you are calm and that you are safe. Whenever the anxiety pops up, just say this affirmation or quote to yourself. This will help you begin to take control of your mind and you will be able to fall asleep.

For those who have a lot of worries, you might need a more involved ritual before bed. One idea is to take the robe or another piece of clothing you're wearing off before you enter the bedroom. This way that piece of clothing is going to hold all of the burdens, but the place of your bedroom is a safe place. Others might like to try other rituals that allow them to release tension in their muscles, e.g. a simple yoga practice. Or you might want to listen to a guided meditation or ambient music to help your brain move into a different energetic pattern before sleep. Try a few things for a week at a time to see what works and then shift it if you're not getting any results. While there are natural supplements you can use to help you sleep, it is often wise to see if you can change your sleep patterns naturally first before moving to medication.

You might also just need to think about how your body works. You may be a person who doesn't need a lot of sleep. Or you might be a person who can't sleep until later into the night. Follow the rhythms that seem to work for you already, tweak them to be better, and see what happens. If you don't feel you're getting the rest you need, perhaps try something different.

But you know your body and you may just need a few nighttime rituals of releasing more than you might need a new bedtime -- or another hour of sleep.

If you do lose sleep and you continue to lose sleep, science does seem to show you can't make that sleep up on a day off or a weekend. The best thing to do is to try to get back on a schedule that feels good for your body as soon as you can. Try to get the sleep you can get when you can get it, but finding a routine should be the goal.

Naps are very helpful in times when you can't get enough sleep. The standard advice, however, is to limit the time to about 20 minutes and at least 3 to 4 hours before your natural bedtime would be. Sleep is not only the place for repairing your body, but it is also the time for dreams and integration. When you make the time for sleep and for deep sleep, you will allow your entire being to be more energized and supported.

Play

Sometimes, all of the advice about taking care of our bodies can feel like work, so it is important to note that play is just as helpful as charting your food and sleep patterns. When we take the time to bring joy into our days, we allow our brains a chance to seek out pleasure and to continuously seek out wonder. We need a break from the everyday lists and the everyday schedules where we can just be silly and unproductive.

This might be difficult to bring into being at first since we're not conditioned to add play into our lives as adults. We're often told it is unnecessary and wasteful when there are THINGS TO DO. But this is a thing to do too. Play allows us to restore ourselves. It allows us to feel happiness and it can be a time of connection with others. We might go play a game indoors, head outside to a basketball court, or wander around a toy store.

Play might look like drawing or coloring in a book. It could look like singing as loudly as you can to a favorite album. It might look like heading to a circus or watching a funny movie. When we give ourselves moments to play, we give ourselves a breath into our energetic selves. We give our worries a rest. They can wait on the sidelines until we're done having fun. And we can come back to the problems refreshed and renewed. We can come back with our nervous systems more regulated and resilient.

Our bodies and hearts require moments when things aren't as serious. Whether we spend five minute or five hours is less of the question, but rather we should ask ourselves if we are making any time at all for things others might find frivolous. If you've neglected your fun time, your play time, it's wise to schedule it in your calendar, just as you would a doctor appointment or some other necessary meeting. Make the time in your schedule and guard it carefully. When you do, you will allow yourself the chance to restore your mind and body.

When you overschedule yourself or when you have to push back playtime, remember that it's not a bad thing to have moments of mistakes or missteps. Rather, we can look at what we have chosen to do and we can decide what might be a better choice later. Or perhaps we can push aside the responsibilities we think are so important and we can escape for just five minutes of play. Give yourself the gift of being like a child again, a child who did things because they were interesting or they seemed like they could be fun.

In some spiritual groups, it is said that there is a childlike soul or energy within all of us. When it does not get attention, it can get cranky. Just as we might become less than ideal versions of ourselves when we're not taking care of ourselves, we need to take care of that inner child. We need to take care of that part of ourselves that still knows what it's like to be in awe of the world. The inner child that knows what it's like to be carefree and in alignment with what's really important -- versus what adult life has told us is important.

It is wise to step in and ask your child self, what do you need? What do you want? What could I do for you? What could I offer you to help you have fun? And when you answer the child inside of you, you will be rewarded with energy and aliveness. You will be able to feel the way you felt when you were just entering the world -- as though anything were possible. Come back to that part of you. Take care of that part of you.

* * *

The body is the foundation upon which your growth and vitality rests. When the foundation is missing a post at the base or it's built on things that aren't permanent, that's when you can begin to feel the shaking and shifting of the structure.

We will all make promises and we might also make mistakes. We will not be perfect in the way we show up for ourselves. But this relationship to your body is the most important one you can cultivate. When your body and mind know you will do your very best for them, you will get returns as well. You can know and honor your body in the present moments you experience. You will be present and alive for the moments you used to take for granted. You will be healthy and well, and you will be able to face things with more ease, more grace, and more resilience.

Settling Your Mind

"The mind is a terrible thing to waste," said Arthur Fletcher. And while we might know this and we have almost certainly heard this phrase, it's not as simple to understand as an action step. We might think of the mind as something that's supposed to work when we're awake and alive, but that will stop working when we are asleep or dead.

But the mind is not an 'on' and 'off' machine. The mind is constantly processing ideas and information we gather from the world around us. It is taking in new things and it is translating them into reactions. Our mind learns how to function from the way others around us have told us to relate, and our mind adjusts based on our habits and our decisions.

It is no surprise that many still think of the brain and the mind as being some of the most mysterious places. Just as soon as you figure out what your brain does in a certain situation, you can also find it reacting in a way that is less than helpful. The brain changes. The brain adapts. And the brain is constantly adjusting. While this might sometimes mean the brain is a frustrating place to live in, it can also be a place of great hope and understanding. It can be a place where we can move things around to make it more effective for our needs. We can change old patterns and introduce new ideas. We can change our minds.

But just as with anything we want to change, it might be something that we don't understand. After all, in a world that's so loud sometimes, we might have trouble hearing what our mind is telling us. Or we might ignore it because we are told to do something differently. Let's settle all of these thoughts -- and the ones that come next.

Why We're Stuck in Our Minds

Our minds are wondrous and perilous at the same time. Since

our brains are always taking in new information, this means there are always new things to consider and to think about in our lives. And depending on what's most important to us or depending on what's most dangerous, we will focus in one or another direction.

But have you ever felt stuck in your mind? Have you ever felt trapped by your thoughts? Most people have. Most people have had days, hours, weeks, or years where their minds have given them so much information that they don't know what to do with it or if they should do anything with it. With all of the mental clutter, how can you truly figure out what's important?

It sounds like it should be easy, after all. Since the thoughts are in your mind, your brain should be able to filter things in a way that will help your understanding and inform your actions. But there are outside forces at play too.

- People we love - From the time we are young, we are taught that things are a certain way. This might not be the truth, but as children and younger beings, we trust the information we receive. We have no reason to believe what we learn to be false. We take in the way that people in our lives think. We try out their ways of relating and we see how they give us the results we want (or not). And even if these ways of thinking are less than productive, they are also habit forming. We can get stuck because *it's the way things have always been done.*
- People we know - Outside of the people that make up our family or close friends, we also are impacted by those who have their own opinions. People tend to want to do things because other people do things. And this influences the way your mind operates. You may not even realize it, but when you're in a group of people and someone talks about a subject in a certain way, you may simply agree with the logic because it makes sense at the time -- or you may not

want to disagree. And over time, being with people who think a certain way can impact the way you interact too.

- Societal expectations - There are messages all around us about how to think, how to behave, what is important, etc. And even though we might know these messages are outside of us, they can get into our psyches. We can begin to assimilate ourselves into society without realizing it. You might notice this the most if you've been able to travel outside of your home country. Things you have assumed to be true may not be true elsewhere. And it can be upsetting, even, since it seems like you might have been thinking incorrectly. No one likes to experience that. Society offers us the 'right' way to think and the 'right' way to use our minds. But are these ideas really the right ways?
- Physical discomfort - Our minds can also be influenced by the way our bodies feel. When we are unhealthy or in pain, we can begin to believe certain things. We can begin to think the world is like _________ because of the way we feel. If our bodies feel stuck, our minds can become stuck too.
- Long-term stress - Those who are under significant stress for long periods of time can also have troubles with settling their minds. Remember a time when you were stressed out and how it influenced your actions. You may have found that you had trouble concentrating or you prioritized things differently than you may have in other times of your life. The stress makes things feel more heightened, and it can make things that aren't that important feel WAY MORE IMPORTANT.
- Trauma - Like long-term stress, having experiences of trauma in your life can also change the way your mind works. You may have different reactions to things than you may have had otherwise. For example, people who have experienced significant loss will often have trouble

letting go of things in their lives. They might also try to make everything important because they want to avoid future pain and loss.

There are many ways in which the overactivity of your mind might not be your fault. You may simply have been influenced by others or by events. However, if the mind can be impacted by things in a negative way, this also means it can be impacted by positive changes and events.

At this moment, are you willing to try something new? Have you felt that things you've thought are not helping you? What do you think? Why do you think? Do you even know anymore?

The Addiction of Thinking and Ruminating

At the core of our bodies is the animal experience. We are designed to react in response to the world around us. When ________ happens, we __________. And the more we do these things and react in these ways, the more these responses become habits. They become the sum of who we are.

If you're a person who finds they have a lot of thoughts at any given moment, I invite you to stop for just a minute. Think about what might happen if you weren't thinking about everything all the time. What would happen for you? How would this feel for you? What might you have in your life that you don't have right now?

Beyond thinking about how things might be better, stop and think about why your thoughts are taking over your life right now. Are you in a period of stress? Are you in a situation that needs a solution? Are you replacing action with thinking about action?

The truth is that we are addicted to thinking much of the time. This is something that we do because we are wired to do it, but also because when we think, it feels like we're doing something. It can feel as though the more thinking we do, the closer we will come to an answer. The more thinking we engage in, the more we will become smarter or wiser or somehow closer to peace. And this often makes sense because when we do think hard about something, it can be a productive process.

But when your thoughts are keeping you up, when your thoughts are causing you to miss out on the moment right now, it's time to break the cycle. It's time to break the addiction of thinking and ruminating. To help break this cycle, it is wise to find a way to slow things down in your brain. This might look like starting with caring for your body and then moving into a place of caring for your mind. By taking a few minutes at the start or end of each day to write down the things you think, you can begin to see patterns and you can begin to see where you might be stuck.

But even before this, we need to cultivate the practice of presence. Perhaps this is the moment where things will change for you. And how can you arrive in this present moment?

Breathe
Notice
Affirmation
Breathe
Repeat until…

Here is a practice to bring you back to this moment where your thoughts can settle or fall away.

You might choose to record this on your phone or other recording device and then listen to it when you need to come back to the present moment.

Take a breath. Allow the air to fill your lungs each time you breathe in and feel the release of tension each time you exhale. Whenever you find a thought coming into your mind, release it with the breath. You don't need to judge the fact that you think. It's natural and it's fine.

But maybe for this moment, you can release the need to think. You can let the thoughts fade away and move outward with your breath. Even if they come back, you can easily release them again.

Allow your inner self to become still and grounded. It can help to picture a root dropping down from the center of your body or from your tailbone or from another place that makes sense to you. Let the root drop down deep enough to connect with the earth, to the place of stillness and nourishment.

As the root deepens into the ground, you can feel yourself becoming stronger and more settled. You have an ally in the earth. You have a support system that you can tap into at any time. All you need to do is drop your roots deeper and connect.

Allow yourself to stay in the deeply connected space where only what is happening in this moment matters.

And right now, you are calm, you are safe, and you are supported.

You are calm, you are safe, and you are supported.

You are calm, you are safe, and you are supported.

Once you feel this fill your bones and your muscles, begin to become aware of the room around you again. You might open up your ears to hear what sounds are emerging. You might smell the air to see what you can smell. You might move your body and touch your fingers. Slowly open your eyes to come back to the place you are.

The mind is like a muscle. It needs to be trained to come back to the present moment when it is out of practice. This might take weeks or months, depending on the way your brain works and depending on how much you return to this practice. I encourage you to try to come back to the present moment as often as possible, perhaps at least once a day until it becomes easier to settle the wandering of your mind.

You can also come up with another script that works better for you. Some find they need different imagery or a longer time to settle down -- all of that is perfect. You are empowered to choose what works best for you.

Releasing Old Thoughts

For many who are looking to settle the minds, it can seem as though they are entering a room with too many pieces of furniture. All of those pieces were purchased with a clear purpose, but now the purpose is less than clear and the room has become cluttered. Old thoughts are the fragments of the past. Some might still inform where we are today, but they might also keep us stuck in a past that no longer exists or that cannot be changed. Just as you need to clear out your home from time to time, releasing old thoughts can help you make room for what is important right now.

Let's take a moment to look around at the room you have created in your mind. What is there that no longer needs to be there? When I'm leading people through guided meditations and trances, I often will ask that people let go and release that which doesn't need to be there anymore. I do this to help folks realize that even if things seem as though they're important in one moment, those same thoughts might be trash later on.

- What thoughts are present in your mind?
- What thoughts keep coming back?
- What thoughts make you feel happy?
- What thoughts make you feel stuck?
- What thoughts are helping you?
- What thoughts are hurting you?
- What thoughts are making you feel less than?
- What thoughts are allowing you to get what you want in life?
- What thoughts do you prioritize?

Examining your mind by thinking about it might seem

contradictory. After all, if we're trying to release the thoughts, we should just stop thinking, right? While learning to become present and unattached to your thoughts is a great help, we also need to know what is coming back again and again. Because when thoughts continue to return, it's because they're not feeling tended to or seen. These thoughts come back because they start a loop of awareness that isn't changed.

For some people, it can be helpful to track the thoughts they have on a particular day or days. When taking the time to write down all of the thoughts you have daily, you are likely to be surprised by how often you are writing things down. You might write down several things each hour or each minute. What you will also notice is that the more you track your thoughts, the more you will start to ask if you need to concentrate on that thought right now. (Or if it's worth thinking about as you don't want to write it down.)

Once you have a sense of how much you think every day -- for better or for worse -- you can begin to see what you want to release. There might be a certain memory or a certain feeling you come back to often. While it's not possible to release what has happened to us, we can release the hold it has over us. We can release the way something interrupts our life and the way it interrupts the momentum of our life.

We can release the power the thought has over us. There are many ways in which we might release the thoughts that hold us back, or at least begin to loosen the hold they have over us. Though you might find you have to do these rituals more than once until you feel released.

But I encourage you to try them:

- Fire - If you're a person who likes to see things in the physical realm, you might want to write out the thoughts that hold you back. You can write them down on a piece of paper or on a bay leaf. Write out what you want to let go of and then burn the item, watching it dissipate until it no longer has power over you. You might choose to do this daily until you feel things loosen.

- Water - You can also choose to cleanse yourself of the thoughts that hold you back. You can have a bowl of salt water in your home or office. Every time you have a thought come back to you, wash your hands or your heart or another area of your body where the thought lives. When you do this, you can know the energy is going into the salt water to be purified and transformed.
- Prayer - For those who feel connected to a god, praying to this being can be helpful. You can sit with the one you believe in and ask them to take the thought away from you. Or you can ask the being to give you information on how to release the thought from your life. You can also just sit and tell the being why you want that thought out of your mind. This sacred time can help you let go and surrender to divine wisdom.
- Gratitude - Another practice that can help you release unwanted thoughts is gratitude. Though we are often taught that negative thoughts are bad, they are things we thought because they made sense at the time. When we instantly avoid them or label them, we can cause them to return all the more ferociously. They can come back with reinforcement, so to speak. They want to be heard, after all. For the thoughts that seem to be more difficult to release or to understand, I encourage a practice of gratitude. Stop and think on the thought you want to release. Think about what it allowed you to have in your life and how it helped you. It might be that a thought about how to live your life kept you in a relationship you valued. Thank you, thought. The thought may have helped to protect you from a certain situation. Thank you, thought. Try to find a way to give thanks for what the thought gave to you and

let it know you learned and that the thought can travel on to someone else.

- Forgiveness - It can be hard to release old ways of thinking when blame is involved. When we feel that someone did wrong to us, we want them to be sorry. We want them to change the way they acted. We want them to take responsibility. But this is not always possible. Sometimes, we are left with just the thoughts circling around our head. We are left with a number of 'what ifs' that may never be settled. And these situations get stuck in our brains. We are stuck with playing out the thoughts again and again. Instead of getting caught up in this cycle, we can begin a practice of forgiving the other person. This might be as simple as pretending to see them and saying, "I forgive you" to the image in your mind. Repeat this process again and again until you begin to feel compassion for this being. You might even find compassion for the choices they made because they were the right choices for them in the moment. And you can then let the thoughts go. You can let them settle and be quieter. But it's not just the act of forgiving someone else that can help. So often we can get caught up in the idea that we should have done better or done differently. We can get stuck in the feeling that if we'd known better, we could have done something else - even when we did the best we could with the information we had. So, we can choose to forgive ourselves. We can look at our own reflections in a mirror and tell ourselves that we forgive ourselves. We can repeat this again and again until we believe it.

There are many ways to release the old thoughts or the repeating thoughts in our minds. We might find we need to use more than one technique. We might find we need to repeat actions again and again. We might find some thoughts need more care and attention than others. And you may find that some thoughts are easily swept out of the room of your mind.

Tracking Your Patterns

With the excavation of thoughts, you may begin to see patterns that repeat. You might find that you always __________ when someone _____________. Or you might notice you end up in the same places more often than you'd like. The body and the mind like to do things without a lot of additional energy. The easiest way is the way they want to take, so they're more likely to default to patterns before trying something new. It's just more efficient. We all have patterns we follow, even if they don't help. Even if they don't support our bigger goals. However, when our minds are busy and cluttered, we might not notice the patterns. Or we might notice the patterns and we might not do anything about it. Let's look at patterns. Let's look at the way we already operate in the world.

I invite you to think about a time in your life that was challenging (not the most traumatic moment of your life, please). Think about a time when something wasn't resolved and a time that still comes into your mind as an unwanted thought. If you're like most people, you will want to think about this story with all of its emotional content and all of the things you've learned about the story since it happened. You will want to think about why it's so horrible and why it continues to fill your mind.

But let's try something new. Instead of looking at the story from the inside, let's look at the story from the outside. Look at the story as though you were someone observing it. Stop and think about what happened in the story, without assigning meaning or blame. What happened? A person did _________ and then this happened ___________. Report on the story as though you were a journalist who was trying to report a story.

Talk about the facts, not the interpretation. When you focus on the facts, you can begin to understand that the story is only as powerful as the meaning you make of it. This is not to discount trauma or the very real pain that may have resulted. All of these things are true too. But when a story continues to hurt you and to interrupt the way your life is unfolding, you can also try to loosen its impact through detached observation. This is much the way that meditation works. We are never going to get rid of the thoughts we have or the things we ruminate on. But we can train ourselves to stop attaching pain to the stories. We can step back and look at things just as they are or were.

We can release the hold they have over us by looking at the facts. And once the facts are clear, then you can move into letting that story go. You can tell the story differently in your mind, which can help it become less powerful as well. Rewrite the story so you're not the victim anymore. You were a part of that story, to be sure, but you don't have to be the one that suffers because of it.

Seeing Your Stories

One of the ways to see your stories is to write them out, but you can also work with some trusted friends to help you see what needs to be seen. One practice comes from the Theater of the Oppressed, created by Augusto Boal. In this exercise, you need a few people to help, or you can step into the different roles on your own. What you need to do is to have the story you want to rewrite or rework and clearly explain it to everyone who is helping you. Each person will take on a different character in the story and they will act it out for you to watch, as though you were the director of a movie. (If you are doing this practice on your own, you can step into each role and act as that person may have acted.)

You can use this exercise to visualize the events as they happened or you can use this exercise to get new information and write a new story. Once you have viewed the story as it happened, you might write down the things you noticed. Or you might ask the 'actors' what they noticed when they were acting things out. You might also ask the 'actors' to continue to interact without any direction about what happens next. They might move to a conclusion that is easier for you to take in. Or you might find the 'actors' guessed at the outcome of the interactions without any direction from you. Another way to use this exercise is to direct the 'actors' to make the decisions you wish the 'real' people would have made. By watching the story play out in the way you wanted it to, this might give you the resolution you need for thoughts that don't seem to go away.

This practice is one that can help you bring your stories to life and into the reality of the present, while offering you control. You can change things, you can stop things, and you can find new ways to think about these parts of your life.

Meditation

While we have already talked about meditation, its importance cannot be stressed enough. This action is crucial for settling your mind. Without a near-daily practice of calming your brain down, your brain will likely wander off more than you'd like. But let's talk about a different kind of meditation that you might be able to do when you're moving during your day. Coming back to your mind and coming back to your thoughts is not about escaping them completely. It is about finding a way to detach from them and to come back to the present. You need to come back to the moment you can control.

To settle your mind, you don't need to be quiet and sit with your legs crossed. Instead, you can move your body and find a way to be present here. For some, this practice might be a little more challenging. We are so often taught to ignore our body or give it things to dull pain. And in doing so, we make it impossible to remember how to be clearly present with our present feelings. You might decide to walk in a park or on a trail or around your neighborhood. No matter what you choose, find a place where you can be safe as you move around. (If you are unable to move your body for a long walk, you can also choose to move around a setting in your mind. Just allow yourself to deepen into an experience of a natural setting that is visceral and easy for you to imagine.)

As you move your body or your mind, allow each step to be a way to ground and calm your thoughts. You can imagine your thoughts moving out of your mind and into the ground beneath you. Let them go, let them go, let them go.

To come into the present moment, look around you. What do you notice? What do you sense? What surprises you? What makes you smile? Become completely present in what is already happening around you. When you find your thoughts trying to go into past stories or future To Do lists, simply take a breath, send those thoughts down into the ground.

With each step, begin to notice more around you and as you do this, begin to feel the way your feet touch the ground. How do you walk? How do you step on the ground? This is not a practice of trying to fix anything, but rather a practice of discovering what you already do. How do you hold your arms? What do your shoulders do? What do your lungs feel like? What do you feel on the skin that's exposed to the outside world? Take a moment to scan your body to see what you feel and what you experience. Think about the experience of muscle and bone. Notice how you have stories that reside in the way you move, and let them go.

Allow your body to tell you what it knows, what it feels, and what it might need. Stay with this experience for as long as you can, slowly building up to longer periods of time as you can. This will help you bring your body and mind back to the present moment, where things are safe. We all just want safety and comfort. We often stay scattered in our minds to avoid feelings that oppose these desires. We want to feel good, dammit, and that means we will do anything to avoid bad things.

But when we can come back into the present moment, we can also feel good. We can remind ourselves that most of the time, we are already safe. And we are in control of making ourselves comfortable. Bring yourself back to yourself. Again and again. And like a snow globe, you can learn to stop and let the flakes fall to the bottom. They can stay there until the next thing shakes us up...and we can go back to settling to the bottom again.

When a Therapist is Needed

With all of this advice and all of these possibilities, you might still encounter unwanted thoughts. You might encounter thoughts that upset you and worry you. You may still encounter thoughts that make you stay up at night -- even if you meditate and detach from the stories in your mind.

When you begin to notice all of these practices are not changing the way you feel, or you notice that you have thoughts that don't seem to make sense, it might be wise to work with a professional to help you calm things down. Most of the time, your mind just needs a little more attention to settle down, but if you've tried these ideas, it might be time for someone else to step in to support you.

The mind is a precious part of you. It can help you become more aware and more empowered in your own life. It can help you feel more alive and interact in more positive ways. Your mind can also have slight imbalances that meditation might be able to help, but not stop. If you have had mental health support in the past, it might be wise to return to this support system again if you find your mind unable (or unwilling) to settle down.

Other signs you need a therapist:

- Others in your life suggest it - Though you might not want this advice from people you love, they often give this advice when we most need to hear it. They are able to look at what is happening to you from the outside and are often more objective than we can be.

- You can't settle your brain - If you have tried meditation, writing, and exercising for at least a week or two, and the thoughts keep coming back, you may want to find a therapist.
- You can't settle down, period - When you notice you have really intense periods of energy and enthusiasm that feel uncontrollable, this can be a sign you need more mental health help.
- You can't cheer up - Conversely, if you notice your thoughts are dark and veering into suicidal, you need to find a therapist. Your mind can begin to tell you things that aren't true when you're feeling low. And when you feel low, you might feel as though things will never get better. They will. You just might need someone else to help you get out of this feeling.

There is nothing wrong with having a therapist help you with the tough times in your life. They can bring you out of your blues or your confusion more quickly. And if therapy is out of your budget, there are often low-cost mental health services available via mobile phone applications and websites. There are also toll-free numbers to call if you have suicidal thoughts and need someone to help you immediately.

* * *

The mind is a place you have made a home for the stories of your life. While these stories may not all be positive, these thoughts are making up who you are at this point. They are a part of your journey to health and well-being. When you can create a healthier relationship to your thinking patterns and your stories, you can become more alive and vibrant. When you take control of your thinking, it will not be able to take control of you.

By working on your body and mind, again, you are creating a solid foundation for your life and for the future that is unfolding before you. The two work together. And as we bring in more actions to support our spiritual life, we will become all the more stable in our being.

Activating Your Spiritual Practice

It's common today to hear that people are spiritual and not religious, as though one is better than the other -- or as though one is deeper than another. No matter how you identify in your spiritual life, science has shown that having a spiritual practice can be just as important as eating well or meditating. When we can connect to something that is bigger than us, it creates perspective and it allows us to cultivate well-being.

No matter if you have walked away from your spiritual practice or if you have never had one before, there are some simple things you can do to activate the possibility that you don't have to do this thing called life on your own.

Daily Practice

One of the things that allows us to come back to ourselves and to our spirit is daily practice. This is simply a routine that we show up for each day, allowing ourselves to have a safe space to return, even when all is falling apart. The key with a daily practice is that it needs to be simple enough to do no matter where you are. It needs to be something you can replicate every single day, even if it doesn't look the same. Let's unpack that a bit. A daily practice works well when there are a few parts:

- Movement
- Silence
- Prayer / Devotion

This doesn't mean your daily practice needs to be long either. You can find a way to make this quick and simple for days when you don't have a lot of time. And you can extend things if you need a little more support on a particular day. You can also shift the order, depending on how things feel to you. You might choose from this menu to help you start:

- Movement - yoga, running, walking, dancing to music, etc.
- Silence - a certain period of time when you simply listen and are present in a moment; meditation.
- Prayer / Devotion - a simple prayer that feels good for you; a song for your spirit; a reading from a spiritual book and contemplation of that reading.

Find a daily practice schedule that works for you. Ideally, the morning time can be easier since you will be able to get the practice done before the rest of your day interrupts the way things are supposed to work. You can also make this more of a ritual by lighting a candle at the start and blowing it out at the end, for example. Or you might have a certain playlist you turn on at the start and then turn off at the end.

It can help to do your daily practice in private, as well as in the same place to make the connection between that place and the daily commitment. I find that I need to set an alarm on my phone to remind me to do my daily practice. While I do it without needing to be reminded, it helps to see it every day. It helps me remember that I made a promise to myself to take this time. I also have a calendar where I check off that I have completed my daily practice. I want to get that check mark, so I show up more often than not.

When you are starting a daily practice, it can be easy to think that skipping one day means you will see no benefits. It's easy to say that you have failed when you do not do your daily practice every day. It's easy to just keep skipping it because you have already interrupted the flow. But let's look at the phrase -- it's daily PRACTICE, not daily perfection. It's about showing up for yourself, most of the time. You will have times when you skip the practice. You might travel and need to skip things. You might be sick one day or you might sleep in. Or you might say to yourself that you don't want to do a daily practice one day. All of these are fine. You are in choice all the time. But if you find you're skipping your daily practice more often than not, here are some things to help you get back on track or back to where you want to be:

- Try shortening your daily practice to get more consistent.
- Reward yourself for sticking to your practice.
- Move your practice to another time of day.
- Get an accountability buddy and check in with them about daily practice.
- Switch up the things you're doing in your daily practice.
- Try a new location for your daily practice.
- Give yourself some guilt-free time off.

You will find a daily practice that is easy to stick to and one that brings you back to your center. In the world you need a place where you can be fully present for yourself. This is where daily practice is essential:

- When things are falling apart around you, go to your daily practice.
- When things are wonderful, go to your daily practice.
- When things are confusing, go to your daily practice.

As your life unfolds and reveals itself to you, daily practice will bring you back to your centered self. No matter how unstable you might feel and no matter what others might do or say to you, you can come back to you. Again and again, imperfectly.

"Come, come, whoever you are.
Wanderer, worshiper, lover of leaving.
It doesn't matter.
Ours is not a caravan of despair.

Come, even if you have broken your vows a thousand times.
Come, yet again, come, come."
Rumi

If you find yourself struggling a lot with daily practice, it can help to check in about what you're doing and whether it's serving you. When we do things because we 'should', it can cause us to be resentful about the practice and the promise we're making to ourselves. Instead, you might want to check in with your body and your schedule. Here are some ways to come back to daily practice when it seems to be falling to the wayside:

- Make it shorter - If you notice you are unable to do all of the things you want to do in your practice, perhaps take away a few things that aren't as much fun or as joyous as you want them to be. Try condensing your daily practice to a few minutes and then expand it on the days when you can do more than that. A daily practice isn't about the length of time you spend, as it's more about the value of the time you spend -- and how often you come back.
- Track your progress - For those who like to see progress, you can also use stickers or some other signal on a calendar to show when you completed your practice for the day. Perhaps when you get to a certain number, you might reward yourself. Or perhaps just seeing that you've been on a streak for a while will help you stay on the streak for longer.
- Step away from it completely - At times, you might need to get away from your practice completely. It might be that life is too much or you're burnt out. Or you just need a break from something. Make this a predetermined length of time and then check back in with yourself about how your life changed because of not doing your practice.

You are allowed to fall away and to come back. In the end, the only person who is impacted by your daily practice is you. (Though others might notice when you have been consistent with it.)

Listening to Spirit

No matter how you define or experience spirit, you can listen. No matter if you've decided spirit looks like a human or that spirit is your favorite tree, listening can help you come to health and well-being. We can listen with our hearts and with our bodies. We can listen with our prayers and we can listen in silence. But we need to listen.

If there are any messages that come up most frequently during spiritual practice, it's that listening is the key to understanding. And when we listen to spirit, it's less about understanding spirit, but more about understanding our relationship to spirit -- and thus, how we understand ourselves. For we are spirit too. We are divine too.

To listen to spirit, I invite you to think about ways you already experience awe and wonder. This might be the time you spend at the ocean or in the woods or with your children. It might be the time you spent at a piano or singing to the radio in your car. It might be the time you spend in a yoga class or the time you spend running until you can't breathe easily. Find the moments that feel good to you, where you connect to something greater. You might find this in your spiritual community or in a book club. Whatever works for you. No matter what it looks like, there is certainly a place for you to be with to listen to spirit.

In these moments and experiences, stop and be present. Let go of any attempts to be 'good' in your listening. Just show up and be where you are. You might do this by looking out and up. You might do this by engaging all of your senses.

You might show up by laughing or crying.

You might show up with questions.
You might show up with worries.
You might show up with wonder.

In these moments, seek to listen between the experiences you have. You may not hear words. You may not understand what you are hearing. You may just walk away with a feeling of connection. You may walk away with a feeling of understanding. You may walk away knowing that you are not alone and that the world is filled with beauty beyond beauty. Because you listened. Because you stayed still long enough to become a part of the awe you experienced.

Look at the stars.
Look at the moon.
Look at a sunrise or sunset.

And listen. There is great wisdom in things that don't always speak to us with words. If only we'd listen more, I hear them say. If only we'd remember we're not as far away from the divine as we've been led to think.

Identifying Your Divine

There have been many conversations (and arguments) about the possibility that humans are just as divine as gods. While you will need to answer that quandary for yourself, I want to offer the possibility that you are just as much a god as a god is.

You are divine. You are blessed. You are spirit and supernatural. And when you can claim these things to be true, you can step into power. You can step fully into yourself. After all, what harm would it be to start worshipping yourself? What trouble would it be for you to see yourself as wise and wondrous? Because the truth is that you are the one who knows best what to do for yourself. You are the one who knows what you believe, what you can believe in, and how you can bring yourself back to balance.

It just feels harder when you have to make the changes yourself. It just feels more difficult when you are the one who has to see the results of your efforts -- or the lack of results. You are a divine being. While you may not be able to change the weather or move mountains, you are a person who can change the direction of your life. And it begins with your mind and your belief in yourself. If you don't believe in yourself right now, I invite you to try anyway. If you don't think of yourself as divine, I invite you to look back at your life to name what you have created. If you don't want to believe you have power, I invite you to consider all those who love you for who you are and not what you do for them. You are divine. And once you begin to believe in this (even if it's not a big belief), you will begin to take hold of the things you want in your life -- and believe you deserve them.

* * *

The mind is the place of creation and birth. It is the place where we sow the seeds of possibility and where we allow dreams to fade. When we can settle the mind into a place of stillness, we can open up places that are ripe with potential. We can invite in the things we really want and desire. So, think of the way that you hold your thoughts. And consider the way you hold onto thoughts that don't serve you as they were designed to.

You can release those thoughts into the world and their energy can fuel something else. They can be transmuted and transformed into motivation for more. They can be removed as obstacles and turned into reminders of how far you've come. The truth is that stories inform us, inspire us, and shape us. When we begin to take up the pen and realize we are the storytellers, we can remember that we are the divine creators. All of the words are spells. All of our thoughts are magic. What will you do to manifest what is truly yours to have?

The Myth of Balance

When it comes to creating something new in your life, you may have turned to other sources of knowledge. And more often than not, there is a pervading message of balance. If you could only get your life into balance, then everything would be fine. If only you could do everything all the time, you would be fine and healthy and happy. But even reading that, I'm sure you realize that this is far from the truth -- and far from reality.

The definition of balance has also been skewed. It sounds today as though it is a static point where you arrive. But in truth, balance is the constant shifting of things to come back to balance. It might be perfectly aligned for a moment, but we have to make choices to come back to what balance looks like for us. And balance might just mean different things in different areas of our lives, in different times of our lives.

Breaking the Definition of Balance

Balance is not a stopping point, but rather a mirage. It looks very real and it appears to be just over the next obstacle...but we will never reach it. We might see it, taste it, understand it, and hope for it, but balance is an idea. When we stop thinking of balance as a perfect place to be, we can release the pressure we put on ourselves to achieve this state. When we stop thinking of balance as something everyone else has but us, we can start to consider how we are out of a balanced state instead of chasing after someone else's balance.

One way to begin to define what balance means to you is to come up with a list of the values you hold to be sacred. What is important to you? From there, you can figure out how to bring these things into your life to foster a sense of balance. To find your values, start by looking at times in your life when you were happy. What were you doing? How were you living your life?

What did you do to support this life? You might also want to look at what you're most proud of in your life. This might be a job or a child or buying your first home. Look back to see what you're proud of in your life, what you're happy you've done and achieved. You might also want to look back for times in your life when you felt content. What was happening at these times? What was NOT happening?

Once you have answered these questions and let them move around in your life, you can look at this list to see what values arise for you as being most important. Ideally, you would choose no more than 10 since you want to focus in on what you value MOST.

Accountability
Accuracy
Achievement
Adventurousness
Altruism
Ambition
Assertiveness
Balance
Belonging
Boldness
Calmness
Carefulness
Challenge
Cheerfulness
Commitment
Community
Compassion
Competitiveness
Consistency
Contentment
Contribution
Control
Cooperation
Correctness
Courtesy
Creativity
Curiosity
Decisiveness
Democraticness
Dependability
Determination
Devoutness
Diligence
Discipline
Discretion
Diversity
Dynamism
Economy
Effectiveness
Efficiency
Elegance
Empathy
Enjoyment
Enthusiasm
Equality
Excellence
Excitement
Expertise
Exploration
Expressiveness
Fairness
Faith
Family
Fidelity
Fitness
Fluency
Focus
Freedom
Fun
Generosity
Goodness
Grace
Growth
Happiness
Hard Work
Health
Holiness
Honesty
Honor
Humility
Impact on Others
Independence
Ingenuity
Inner Harmony
Inquisitiveness
Insightfulness
Intelligence
Intellectual Status
Intuition
Joy
Justice
Leadership
Legacy
Love
Loyalty
Mastery
Merit
Obedience
Openness
Order
Originality
Patriotism
Perfection
Piety
Positivity
Practicality
Preparedness
Professionalism
Prudence
Reliability
Resourcefulness
Restraint
Results-oriented
Rigor
Security
Self-actualization
Self-control
Selflessness
Self-reliance
Sensitivity
Serenity
Service
Shrewdness
Simplicity
Soundness
Speed
Spontaneity
Stability
Strategic
Strength
Structure
Success
Support
Teamwork
Temperance
Thankfulness
Thoroughness
Thoughtfulness

Timeliness
Tolerance
Trustworthiness
Understanding
Uniqueness
Unity
Usefulness
Vision
Vitality

You might also have other words or values to add and to put into your top 10 list. Once you have these values, stop and think about what these mean to you. It can help to clearly define what each of those values might look like out in the world. For example, when you value 'Impact on Others,' you might describe this as having a positive impact on the lives of others. Or you might want it to mean that you have an impact on everyone, whether that is good or bad. In this exercise, you will begin to name what is most important to you. And from there, you can arrange your life in a way that is balanced -- for you.

Finding What Balance Looks Like

To create a picture of a life that is balanced for you, take those words you have defined as being your values. Look at each of these words and examples and see where your life is already matching up to their meaning.

- In what ways are you already living up to these values?
- In what ways are you not living up to these values?

It can help to look at this process as a fact-finding mission versus an evaluation of your life. You are just here to collect information and to find out what needs to shift. You do not need to berate yourself for the ways you haven't been in alignment with your values. You can simply notice what you notice. You can arrive where you are. You can become wiser and more prepared for the life you want to create from where you are right now.

I suggest you write out these values onto a piece of paper. You might choose to decorate it or be creative in your writing. You can also choose to take one piece of paper for each value and make a collage of images that represent its felt sense (a.k.a. the way it feels in your body and mind when you experience it). Put these words and these pictures in places where you can review them often. At this point, it is just about learning and not about changing anything. It is about making sure these are your top values and your top places of focus for the coming days.

Take some time to look at these words and these ideas. See what solutions you already see just from noticing where you are and where you are not. But don't commit to changing or even consider changing anything yet. It takes time to come up with ways to shift your life and the more time you can allow things to simmer in your mind, the more likely you are to find things that will end up being long-term changes instead of quick fixes because you want to do something, even if it's not the right thing to do. You can create a time container in which you think on these values. You might change them up or qualify them more. You might choose new values or spend time journaling about them until you really understand what they mean and what they have to offer you.

I would suggest considering this process over the course of a moon cycle. So, you might sit down and discover the information around the full moon or new moon and then sit with this information until the next full or new moon. In these 28 days, you can think about the ways in which your life is being depleted by the things that don't align (new moon energy) and you can think about the ways in which you have brought your values into practice (full moon energy).

At the end of this moon cycle, you can begin to look at what needs to happen to change things, if you've decided things need to change. As with any life changes, it can help to start small and see how things feel different. For example, if you chose a value that talks about truth, you might choose to be truthful in all of your email communications for a month. This way, you can see what it feels like to live this value before moving onto truthfulness in all of your communication and relationships. Or the time you spent thinking about the ways you need to shift your life may have offered you bigger steps. You are in choice to take those bigger steps too.

To track the progress you've made, it can help at the end of the day to reflect on your actions. You might stand by the list of your values to remind yourself how you aligned with these words that day. If there are ways you did not come into alignment, then you might ask yourself how tomorrow might be better. Think of this as learning and growing and moving toward a state of alignment that is right for you. You will not hit all of your values every day. Or you might align with your values, but it may be sporadic -- this is okay. This is not a practice of perfection, even if that is a value of yours. Perhaps you can reframe that as a desire to do your very best. And to love yourself even if you fall short of these larger expectations.

You can also create a checklist on an application or a piece of paper that lists all of your values. Bring this with you during your day and check things off when you notice you have made a choice that is in alignment. For those who like to see their progress and stay present with their actions, this immediate feedback can be helpful. Or you might choose to share your progress with a loved one. You might ask them if you can check in with them about your values once a week. And they might be inspired to join you in this work too. Together, you can cheer for each other and help each other find solutions for issues as they arise.

This is a journey of finding what balance looks like for you - and only you. This is not a contest to be better than others. In fact, when you begin to feel that this realignment is burdensome and stressful, you may want to stop and take inventory of your motivations. Are you being motivated by wanting a more contented life? Or are you trying to live up to someone else's expectations? You may need to go back to the list of values to see if there are others that fit better for you now . It might be that this is a process of shedding the values of others in order to find out what works for YOU. Perhaps for the first time ever. Your values should be yours and yours alone. Even in your partnerships, you might have shared values, but it is likely you will not have the same list of values.

Recalibrating Your Life

As you begin to bring your life back into alignment with what's true for you, you may find that others aren't as happy as you might become. When you start to create a life that works for you, it upsets the balance of the lives of others. But this doesn't mean you should stop. In fact, when you start to see others in your life become upset with your happiness, it is a sign that you are doing something you have needed to do for a while. Others in your life should be happy to see you grow and seek a better life. They should celebrate you and support you.

Yet, it is hard for others when they see you change. It can mean they have to question their interactions with you. They might need to change the way they relate to you. They might need to change the way they communicate. And it's possible you might lose some people in your life as you live in alignment with your values. They may not be willing to support you or to be on the journey with you. While no one wants to hear that, it is a common occurrence. Throughout the process of finding your health and well-being, you may lose people along the way.

With that in mind, you need to have a practice of self-care to keep yourself in a balanced and aligned state as much as possible. You need to take care of you because no one else will. You need to find out what you need to feel your best and to do your best and to live your best life. Just as with the myth of balance, self-care has also been maligned due to capitalism. And we'll need to undo what you think you already know about this necessity for your health. Self-care is not just the products you buy. It is the act of refilling your cup.

The Truth about Self-Care

Sometimes it can seem that self-care has become a product, a commodity, and even a thing that EVERYONE does. But the truth about self-care is that it is also a sign that your life is out of balance. Having to focus so much on self-care just to keep yourself from falling apart is not a sign of well-being. It is a sign that bigger things need examination.

- Is your life filled with things you want to do?
- Is your schedule able to accommodate down time and free time?

Self-care is not something to be relegated to the one free weekend you have. And it's not something that is all that exciting or sexy or expensive. It is a practice of coming back to yourself, a practice of showing up for yourself when you realize you need more care and attention. And, ideally, self-care is a practice that is in place long before you need it to be.

What Self-Care Is

According to the Oxford dictionary, self-care is *the practice of taking action to preserve or improve one's own health.* When you see this definition, you see that it's not about face masks or about heading to the spa when you're overworked. Originally, self-care was the mindset that your body requires you to take care of it -- for self-preservation. But this isn't supposed to be a reaction. Self-care is meant to be refilling your cup so things never get so low that you become ill or burnt out. In the times we're in, however, it's easy to forget this. When you have twenty things on your To Do list and no time in which to get all of them done, you likely feel that your health is the last thing you should focus on. When you have a job, you can't call in sick to or you need to show up for as many hours as possible, self-care is not a part of your everyday consideration. And honestly, why would it be?

However, with all of the attention self-care gets in the current press and conversation, it's become clear that self-care means something else today. It is used as a 'reward' for working hard or for working too hard. And often, the advice about self-care looks like buying one more thing. It looks like being offered advice about things you can't afford. It looks like perpetuating a cycle -- especially for marginalized groups.

When you are already suffering at the hands of capitalism and commercialism, you don't have time to do more or to buy more. You can get caught in a cycle of not having any way to feel better or to refill your cup. You can't pay people to do your laundry for you. You can't take time off to relax. You have to keep going. You have to keep working.

I wish we could change the current mindset and thinking. Ideally, a systemic and structural change would be best. In lieu of that, we can learn to take care of ourselves in ways that are nourishing -- and that can also be sustainable. After all, you likely know the consequences of not taking care of yourself. You likely have stretched yourself too far and for too long. Most of us have. Most of us have wondered aloud, what could I have done differently to avoid that again?

What Happens without Self-Care

When we're stuck in a life or in a cycle that doesn't allow for focus on our bodies and our minds, we can get depleted. Those who are able to have a basic level of self-care will not hit rock bottom as quickly as those who are constantly fighting to just be okay. To be clear, those who already suffer from busy-ness and unwellness will feel the effects of not having self-care more quickly than those who have resources. A lack of self-care can show up as:

- Being unmotivated - One of the first signs of being out of touch with your needs is feeling that you don't want to do anything that you need to do. You might look at your To Do list and not finish anything or you might move through things so slowly that the list seems longer than it should seem.
- Feeling bored - Even if you love your job or you love school, you might begin to hate what you're doing. You might feel disinterested and unable to remember why you signed up for this thing in the first place.
- Not being able to sleep - Many folks will be unable to slow down their thoughts. They will begin to have trouble either falling asleep or staying asleep. You might notice you can't get to bed at your normal time or you can't stick to a schedule.
- Wanting to sleep all the time - Conversely, and possibly from not being able to sleep, you might want to go to bed all the time. You might start to get to bed earlier than normal or you might start hitting the snooze button more often in the morning. As an escape route, you might turn to sleep to get away from all that stresses you out.
- Appetite changes - Some will find their appetite changes when they're stressed out or not feeling supported. They will stop eating as much or they might start eating more, depending on their coping strategy.
- Lower productivity - If you're feeling low on energy, you might start to notice you can't get as much done during the day. Even outside of your personal To Do list, you might not be able to get to all of the things your work expects you to do. Your co-workers or boss might begin to notice the decrease in your output.
- Anger / despair - And it makes sense that when you don't feel supported that you might begin to feel angry that you have to do so much in the first place. You might begin to

feel as though you're never going to be able to get ahead again or you may never be able to get to a place that feels happy or balanced.

- Sadness / depression - For some, the place of not having enough time to care for yourself can also cause depression. It's sad when you don't feel well and when you don't feel like you have any choice in the matter. You might begin to isolate yourself and you might begin to feel more alone than you are. And this depression can cause you to continue to feel as though taking actions may not be helpful, so you take few actions...and it's a hard momentum to break.
- Loss of purpose and drive - At the very least and yet at the very core, when we don't take care of ourselves, we can begin to lose our very drive for what we want in our lives. We might begin to question why we're doing what we're doing. Once we begin to feel directionless, it can feel as though there might be no purpose in our presence.

As you can see (and possibly relate), taking care of yourself is important to your entire being. It not only impacts the way you feel, but it can also impact the way you feel about yourself. You might begin to feel as though you are someone who is not worth care and support. But there are ways we can break away from these trains of thought. We can get away from these patterns and we can move ourselves into a more supportive practice of care.

However, this is a process that takes more than just a day off. We need to figure out where we can refill our cups. And while we may not be able to escape the lives we have to live and the jobs we have to hold, there are ways to keep ourselves buoyed. As in *The Handmaid's Tale,* "Don't let the bastards get you down." We won't.

Creating a Life that Requires Less Refilling

You may want to start this process of self-care by looking at what makes your cup feel empty. What are the things in your life that seem to stretch you versus support you? While these items might vary based on the day or situation, here are a few examples you might relate to:

- Too many work hours
- Too many deadlines
- Too many tasks
- Too many people asking you for support or help
- Critical people in your life
- Sad people in your life

What makes you feel drained in your life right now? There's a concept in autoimmune disease communities around the spoon theory. This is a theory in which you only have so many spoons in a day. When you use up your spoons, you have no more energy to give. But not everything in your life requires the same number of spoons. And on some days, the spoons you need for a certain task might be more or less. For example, when you have the flu, making breakfast might take up far more spoons than when you are not sick.

Another theory or concept that's emerging is the idea of the fork theory. While most of us can handle stress, when there are too many stressors, it can become unmanageable. Said another way, when we have one fork in our back, we might hurt and be overwhelmed, but it's okay. It will go away. But when we have multiple forks in various parts of our body, we start to hurt too much and things begin to feel untenable.

Thinking about the spoon and fork theory, you can begin to rate your life in terms of the energy things take from you. What makes you feel good? What makes you feel awful? True, we can't necessarily live a life that is perfectly perfect all the time, but the more we can move things into a direction that feels good to us, the more we will enjoy the life we have as a whole.

It might be wise to start a period of self-evaluation. Think about what takes up your energy (a.k.a. Your spoons). Think about what forks are already in your life. When you begin to notice what's true about your life right now, you can begin to see what might need to change. Or what might need to be shifted so it's more comfortable. When you know what doesn't work for you, you can begin to see where you need to make changes to impact your life in positive ways. It would be great to have this be an overnight or instantaneous process, but that's unlikely to happen. (But if it does -- great!)

To create a life that requires less self-care emphasis, we need to look at the life you have and what you need to change. But you also need to look at the things that you want to change and see if you could change them.

Your Ideal Day

A practice I find to be most helpful is to draw up a plan of the way you want your days to look. This is the ideal day, not a shift of your life just yet. Think about what you would want your perfect life to look like. Write out the times that you would wake up, when you would eat, etc. Describe the perfect day for your energy and for your happiness. Get as detailed as possible with each hour of the day. Figure out what you really want and how you want to feel.

Once you have the day described, stop and look at the schedule. What does it make you feel? How does it shift the way you're breathing? Does it fill you with hope or another feeling? As you look at this schedule or vision for your life, what is one thing you could do to change your life right now? Could you shift your schedule so you're waking up at your ideal time? Could you move around your meal times to be in alignment with your vision? Are there little things you could do to make a shift right now?

Nourishing Yourself Each Day

Just as important as what you can bring into each day is what you can remove from your days. As you look at your current schedule, what can you remove to make space for things you really enjoy? If this feels overwhelming, you can start with small steps. You can start with removing 10 minutes of things you don't like to do. For example, if you hate going to do the laundry, can you go with a friend? Can you go to a new laundromat that has better music or is close to a place that you might be able to grab a snack?

Before we move on, I want to be clear that building a life that feels better is not just about becoming an optimist about what is already in front of you. This practice and this journey are about finding a grounded mindset and then living a life from there. When you are in the present moment, you can be clear about what you really want and what sustains you. Nourishing will likely look simple. In contrast to the way magazines and TV shows make self-care sound, the basic things are really all we need to do to make our lives more delightful:

- Eat well
- Move your body
- Get rest
- Stay in contact with friends
- Connect with spirit

Though it might be unexpected, self-care is often very boring. It is a practice of simply showing up to care for yourself in a way that ensures your health and well-being. To nourish ourselves is to make sure we have the essentials. There's a meme online that talks about how humans are basically house plants with more complicated emotions. And that resonates with me. We are animals at our core, with the need for things that make our bodies feel good and well. When we step away from those basic practices, we will not feel well. But when we come back to the basics of life, we will lift the haze of unwellness.

If you find your mind moving to thoughts that these 'basic' things are too simple, give yourself a moment to think about your thinking. Take a breath and see where your body is when you think about giving it more attention. Does it seem to be happy? Hopeful? Encouraging? Do you already give yourself these 'basics' of self-care? Do you already show up for your body and your mind every day? If so, then you may need more. And we'll get to more soon. But if you are in a place where you first want to dismiss any validity of these practices, I might encourage you to try out a few of these actions to see how they make your body feel. While people who sell things want you to believe you need to spend more money on things to practice self-care, you really don't.

Self-care is often so dull in the way that it's just the consistency of practices that are already good for you. There are really no secrets and no hidden mysteries. What is hard is that you do need to make time for the simple, repetitive things. They are not quick fixes and they are not instantly going to help you feel 100% better about everything in your life. But. When you practice the kind of self-care that means showing up for yourself, when you practice the self-care that you don't necessarily share on social media, you begin to show up for what you really need -- versus what others think you need.

It is hard to extract ourselves from the peer pressure of current trends in self-care. We often think we're doing it wrong when we really aren't. We think that because we're not doing what some celebrity says, we're never going to feel as great as they seem to feel. And that's understandable when you hear those sorts of messages over and over.

Yet, you are the one that knows how to nourish yourself best. You are the one who knows what you need, truly. And even if you're out of practice or you're not quite sure what you need today, you can listen to your body. You've already begun to listen more. And the more you practice, the clearer the messages of your body will be.

If you're already feeling overwhelmed by the practice of trying to not feel overwhelmed, then you might want to look at your life and your schedule for 10 minutes a day to do something that makes you feel good. This could be cooking yourself a meal. It could be going for a walk around the block. It could be reading a chapter of an exciting book. It could be something else. But what is the way you can show up for yourself and nourish yourself today? How can you do this every day? How might you be able to bring in more and more attention to yourself each day?

How to Live Your Own Life

You need to live your own life. You need to find out what makes YOU happy. And this means disconnecting from things that might not fill you up. (And to be clear, part of this is remembering that what is nourishing for you might not be nourishing for someone else. This is about tapping into what is true for you, listening, and then taking action.)

Where we might admit it or not, the real life people have an impact on how we live our lives. What people are serving you and helping you be a better person? Who do you look forward to seeing? Who do you avoid seeing if possible? Who makes you smile and feel better about your place in the world? Who makes you wonder if you're doing anything right?

While it's true that our reactions are our own and that people may not be 'trying' to do anything to us, it is also true that we don't have to be around anyone we don't like. Though we may have been taught to try to get people to like us, it's actually the other way around. We should be looking to others and seeing if we like them first. In the practice of learning to live our own lives, we come to places where we need to make decisions. We need to question the way things are working and adjust the things that don't seem to be working. Once you have worked on shifting the way your communities and interactions look online and in real life, stop to assess how things feel with these changes. Are things feeling better? Do you feel more nourished? Do you still feel depleted?

For some, this practice might be challenging as it causes you to see that you may have been immersed in situations that were not healthy for you. And while you could linger in blame and anger at yourself, you can also find ways to thank the ways in which those people offered you insight into what is right for you. And what is not. You may find, in time you can come back to certain people and you might be able to interact in a supportive way online with people that used to bug you. Or you may not. It's up to you.

A few caveats in this discussion include:

Critical thinking - With all of these pieces of advice comes the assumption that you will think critically of the choices you make. You will check in with yourself about why you think the way you do, whether this thinking comes from yourself and experience or from rumor. You will also want to think about the why of what you're doing and whether you are avoiding something that needs to be faced head on.

Opposing thoughts - In a world with people who think differently, we are always going to find people who think the opposite we do. We will find their opinions annoying at times and offensive at others. But hearing opposing thoughts can be helpful in allowing us to see just how much we believe in our own. And hearing another side can also be helpful in understanding someone else, even if we don't agree. Of

course, this doesn't apply in situations where someone's opinion is life-threatening to someone else.
Abusive / harmful situations - When you're in a situation that has included abuse or harm, you don't have to interact with that person ever again. So often, people are told they should give someone another chance, but you don't have to. If you have been harmed, you can simply stay away from them forever. You don't have to forgive anyone. You can walk away.

I bring all of this up because there are ways in which our society can sometimes attempt to shame us out of our sovereignty. We are too often told we don't believe something because no one else does. (They do.) And we are too often told we can't do something because others don't do it. (They do.)

I also find it helpful to disconnect from things that might give you too much information or that might showcase a lifestyle that you can't follow:

- Turn off ads / stay away from commercials
- Get off of social media that's damaging
- Step away from positive posting (sometimes)
- Follow groups and people who uplift you
- Track what makes you feel good vs. what is supposed to make you feel good

It can seem impossible to get away from things that might influence our thinking and our actions. And, honestly, unless you can get away from society as it looks right now, you will still be exposed in some way -- even with this advice.

But it can help to set aside time each week to step away from social media and advertising. You might schedule this time away on your calendar and just turn all of the devices and machines off. You might choose to have whole days of disconnect. Or you might try out small bits of time until you feel more balanced in your use. (Side note: I realize that many people talk about disconnecting from social media altogether in order to be healthier. But many people need social media and other outlets to be connected with people and communities. You know what's best for you. Staying away from what doesn't make you feel good is a better piece of advice.)

Having some disconnect time will allow you to feel less attached to hearing what everyone is saying. And it can help you to stop thinking that what you see is real or the whole story. Most of us don't post things on social media that are negative, after all. So, when we look at social media, we only see a part of the story. We only see what others want us to see. We don't see the negative emotions and the ways in which life doesn't always go the way someone expects it to go. Step away as you can. Gain perspective. Realize that you can also be with yourself in ways you know to be supportive and positive.

Social media can be damaging and upsetting. It can be filled with good news and reminders of what you haven't done yet. It can also be filled with upsetting images and poorly chosen words. It can be a place that feels like a battlefield instead of a supportive community. Some of this is just the way things go when you have a lot of people in one place at the same time. But you might also be able to minimize damage from social media by only connecting with people and groups that feel nourishing to you. Remove the people you barely know or the ones that seem to be in opposition to things you hold to be true.

You don't have to be friends with everyone. You don't need to be the witness to the things others do and say. You can cultivate your own experience in life and decide what's right for you. You can stay away from people who don't support you. You can talk with people who agree with you. You can have a social media experience that is positive and uplifting.

It takes a little work. Some of it is reducing your time online and some of it is only interacting with those who you want to interact with. Start with an inventory of your current experience. Who do you like? Who upsets you? Figure out what you want to do with the folks you don't like and then remove them from your accounts. Or you can usually find a way to 'hide' them so you can still see them if you want to.

And it's not just the negative people that you may want to remove from your life. You might also have people in your life whose positive posts and attitudes might make you feel less about your own choices. This is not to say they're trying to hurt you or to burst you, but you also don't need to have those folks in your view when it doesn't feel good. You might also choose to remove these people from your timelines to see how that makes you feel. It might be really helpful for you to have contact with folks who show the full range of experience, versus just the good things.

Once you have removed or hidden the people that don't seem to help you feel better about yourself, you can begin to introduce groups and people who would make you feel good. Find communities of people like you. Find people who share common interests. Be with people who are likely to 'get' you. Spend more time there. Of course, it's probable that you won't like everyone you find in these groups. There are always some people you will not like -- and you don't have to like everyone. You can simply stay for what serves you.

You are in control of your choices, your feelings, and your experience, for the most part anyway.

Nourishing yourself starts with listening, but also means you do what's right for you -- no matter what anyone else thinks. When you take responsibility for your own feelings and you do not harm anyone in the process, you are the only one that gets to be in the decision-making of your life.

Self-Care Strategies

When you are just realizing how far away you have been from your own self-care, getting started can seem daunting. You might begin to wonder if you will ever be able to take care of yourself the way you deserve to be taken care of. And when you feel behind in your self-care, how do you catch up?

You can just begin where you are. You can begin right now. Find the time that you have and allow it to be yours. Allow this time to be the time you will have to care for yourself. Stop thinking there is a 'right' amount of time. There is the time you have. You can use the time you have:

Get away - If there is a way, get out of the place you are. Literally. Stop what you're doing, drop what you need to do next and get away from your current place. This might look like going for a walk around the block. It might look like hiding in the bathroom for a little while. Do what you need to do to get away from where you are so you can come back to yourself. You don't even have to achieve anything when you leave where you are. You can just leave. Moving out of one physical space to another can be just what you need to feel unstuck.

Bathe / shower - You might also take the time you already spend in the shower or bath to help you connect back into yourself. Spend a little more time washing your hair. Make sure you get soap on every part of your body. Shave things if you want to shave. Use scented things if you have them and want them. Envision the water washing away any tension or stress. Allow your muscles to have a little extra time in hot water or cold water. Be with yourself and no one else. Feel good, feel whole, and feel nourished.

Laugh - When you're feeling down or unmotivated, it can help to shake that feeling by watching a movie or finding a video that makes you laugh. Find something that makes you feel differently, even if the cause of your anxiety doesn't go away. One of the common pieces of advice in therapeutic practices is that you need to get out of your feelings every now and then. It's okay to feel things, but when you get stuck in these feelings, that's where it's not healthy anymore. You can start creating grooves in your emotional landscape that want to stay in certain feelings, and you don't want to be stuck. Redirect your feelings with laughter.

Cry - And for some, letting feelings out is the way to make sure they feel more grounded. You might need to just cry for a while. If you're the type of person who doesn't cry because of a fear they may not stop, you can let that go. You will eventually stop. You will get tired. You will get dehydrated. You will stop. The tears will end. But as long as they need to flow, let them flow. They are healing and recalibrating.

Distract - Beyond laughing and crying, you can find other ways to distract yourself. It is said that it takes about 90 seconds to get unattached to an emotional experience. As long as you can distract yourself for that long, you will be able to stop the feeling from taking over. Another thing to keep in mind is that your body can feel anxiety and panic for only about 20 minutes as you will then run out of adrenaline (and it takes a bit to make more). If you can distract yourself for that amount of time, you can bring yourself back to a more grounded state. This distraction could look like reading, knitting, playing with a pet, calling a friend, or cleaning the bathroom. Do what you can to keep your mind from getting stuck and you will be able to come back to where you are.

Limit - For those with many worries and wonderings, you will find it helpful to limit the worry time. Set aside 10 to 15 minutes a week (yes, a week) to worry. This will help your body know you have time to think about things, but it will also allow you to stay present more often with what's actually happening versus what could happen. Once the time is over, let your brain and body relax. Most worries that do not have clear causes are not things you can fix. And if there are things you can fix; you can take action but you also don't have to worry about them. You can meet them head on, as best you can.

Ground - One of my favorite practices is to ground myself by connecting with the earth. Too often, it's easy to try to connect with things that don't have any stability, e.g. expectations, goals, etc. But the earth is steady and solid (even if it has tectonic plates that shift constantly).

I ground by finding a way to come into contact with the ground. I might take off my shoes and even my socks to touch the floor. Or I might go outside to touch the ground. You can also wear shoes or sandals or socks. Do what works for you.

What is important is to become aware of the way you interact with the earth. Notice the way that you are pulled by gravity and how you rest on the earth. You might close your eyes or you might keep your eyes open. Allow yourself to breathe at a pace that feels nourishing in this moment. You might need longer breaths. You might need more breaths versus longer breaths. Allow your body to tell you. Respond to your body if things change.

Once you have found the breath that makes sense, continue to breathe and become present in the moment you are in. You might start to notice how your body feels and what it needs. You might need to shift your body to feel more comfortable or you might not. You might continue to move your body until you feel completely relaxed. You might dance. You might sway. You might stay as still as possible.

Allow your breath to push down into the ground, helping you feel even more connected. With each breath, imagine being connected more deeply to the layers of the earth. Continue to move down as deeply as you'd like to go. Once you're as deep as you'd like to be, give gratitude for this depth and connection. And then begin to move upward, moving from the place of depth to the place of opening. Focus instead on the breath in and how it pulls you back up through the layers. Bring your awareness up through the body, through the ways that you are and the way your body feels in this moment.

Allow the awareness to rise past your head and into the sky. You can allow your awareness to go as far as the clouds, the atmosphere, the stars, the galaxies, etc. Go as far as you need to go in order to feel connected to all that is above. And when you are connected to that place of expansiveness or openness, you might feel gratitude here. For the divine, to the mystery of places you will likely never see.

Once you are ready, come back down to your body and to the earth, to the place where you are the kiss between earth and sky. Present. Calm. Resourced. If doing a meditation or grounding like this isn't something that feels great to you or it takes up too much of your time, there is another way you can connect back into the earth whenever you like. All this takes is finding an item you can carry with you or wear on you. This might be a stone or a rock, or it might be a necklace or a pair of socks. Choose something that you have around -- no need to spend money or to find something new.

Whenever you have a moment or a day when you feel completely grounded and at peace, take a moment with that item and breathe the feeling into the item. Allow the item to fill up with this feeling so every time you touch it, you can go back to that feeling. You can know that feeling is possible. You can continue to feel that feeling in that moment, even if it's not what you were experiencing.

You can anchor in the experience of grounding into the item, where it can be accessed any time. Some people also find it helpful to anchor a feeling into their body. This might be a place that feels settling on your skin or a place that you normally touch when you're anxious. Instead of feeling anxiety, go back to this spot to feel what it's like to be at peace. Touch that space and imagine the feeling pouring into that area. The feeling stays there and lives there. Whenever you touch that space again, you will tap back into the memory of peace.

The more you can create places of comfort and grounding around you, the more you can bring yourself back, refill your cup and allow your body to feel at home in itself -- without a need for fancy face masks or long baths.

What about Those Face Masks and Baths?

As you've probably already noticed, I am not a fan of the current advice about self-care and about buying things in order to make yourself feel better -- for a moment. And I do use face masks from time to time. And sometimes I do call it self-care. But it's more of a moment of making myself feel special. It is also a distraction. It is also a moment where I can use that time to think about bigger things that need to be changed in my life to make it more sustainable.

There is nothing inherently wrong with a small treat or mask every now and then. There really isn't. You can do as you like and when you like. It is simply worthwhile to look at the 'why' from time to time. Think about why you're doing one thing over another thing.

- Think about why you're not drinking more water or why you're not eating vegetables more often.
- Think about why you're keeping certain people in your life, even though you know they're hurting you on some level.
- Think about why you stay in a job that doesn't serve your bigger goals or dreams.

- Think about why you aren't taking small steps toward making yourself feel nourished.

I can't stress enough that this is not a line of reason that involves judgment. I invite you to explore your life with curiosity. Open up to the wisdom of what is in the present and how it might shift to open to more joy, more vitality, and more resilience. Your life will never be completely perfect. You will likely not have everything you've ever wanted. But when you live your life in awareness of what you need to feel nourished, it won't matter what's missing. You will feel too good to dwell about that.

* * *

Self-care is a tricky business, in many ways. Not only does it ask us why we think we need the self-care in the first place, but it also asks us if we know what it means to truly care for ourselves. Many of us don't know how. Many of us have never been taught how to care for ourselves because we were brought up and were friends with people who were never taught either. So, we go to social media or to magazines for advice. We go outside of our trusted circle to get advice on how to better hold our own bodies and hearts. We need to come back to ourselves. We need to come back to the wisdom of bodies and bones. We need to come back and be quiet enough to realize we already know what we need, even if it seems basic and boring.

We already know that our bodies require certain actions to feel alive and to be alive. We likely already know that our bodies require attention every day, not just when we're sick and not just when we're in pain. Our bodies are longing for us to listen and to hold even when everything seems okay or stable.

I invite you today to take a few moments to care for yourself in the ways you know how. Stop and give yourself a promise to learn how to care better, to love more fiercely, and to be in better relationship with the vessel that holds you -- even when you're hard on it. Care for yourself. Care for your beautiful self. It doesn't have to cost money. It doesn't have to look a certain way. But care for yourself. You deserve it.

Cultivating Resilience / When Things Go Wrong

While it would be great if taking care of ourselves would allow us to avoid pain in our lives, that's not the way it works. You know this and it's still frustrating when it happens. We are not going to get through this life without a difficult event, unless we decide to never take risks, engage with people, or connect deeply with someone. Because we are all going to face troubles and traumas, we will do ourselves a favor by actively seeking out ways to prepare ourselves for the inevitable.

This is not to say that we should become hyper vigilant, nor does this mean that we should simply plan our lives to be painful. Instead, we can cultivate resilience in our lives. We can create a foundation of skills and tools that allow us to come back from the darkest, scariest places. We might come back changed, but we can still come back. We can face hard things, bad things, and unexpected things, and still return to the places of our bodies. Like any skill, we can cultivate our own support and we can build our ability to be resilient.

What Resilience Is / Normalizing Life

According to the Oxford Dictionary, the definition of resilient is to be *able to withstand or recover quickly from difficult conditions.* Like so many other words in the English language, the meaning has been corrupted with the introduction of the internet and of those who wish to make money from normal human experiences.

Resilience is the way that we come back from what has gone wrong. Some might say this implies you are wrong to have gone away from yourself during difficult moments, but this is not the case. When you are resilient, you do not come back to some perfect place. After a traumatic or difficult place, you are not the same person. You know different things. Your experience of the world is going to be different. This is normal. To repeat, this is normal.

When we face things we never thought we'd face, we have reactions and responses we may not have expected. And of course, this happens. For example, if we were to lose someone suddenly in a car accident, we are shocked and angry and sad. We might have months when we feel that everything is okay and manageable and then we simply fall apart. Or some people might never react to the situation at all, carrying on as though nothing happened. Or they might start to blow up at everyone around them because their pain was never seen by others.

No matter why our resilience might be tested, it is necessary to say that being resilient does not come with a grade or a score. There is no perfect way to be resilient, just as there is no perfect way to be traumatized. There is a story that Brene Brown once shared on a radio show about someone who asked her how to raise children who are resilient. And when the parent was asked by Brown what causes resilience, the mother realized that resilience comes from facing hard things and getting through them.

We become resilient because we have practice. We are resilient because things happen that we could never expect and never wish on anyone. We face them. We experience them. We hate them and we grow because of them. We may still have grown without these experiences, to be sure. But with these experiences, we are able to become something more than we were before. We are flexible and we can bounce back. We can have feelings and reactions and we come back to ourselves. Perhaps we come back a little more tired or anxious about life. Perhaps we come back proud of our ability to return at all. But we come back. More often than not, we come back.

And it is normal to worry you will not. It is normal to wonder if you can come back, if you truly are as resilient as life seems to ask us to be. As resilient as life seems to require we be. We face sickness, deaths, unexpected accidents, losses, and betrayals. We come up against situations we never thought we'd face. We come up against problems we can't solve and worries we can't halt. But we still have things to do and people to love. We still have work and homes and bills. The world doesn't stop because we are upset and aching. The world doesn't slow down because we need it do -- and we might really need it to.

In a world where the next day seems to offer even more absurdities from governments and people in our lives, resilience is a trait that we not only need to cultivate, but we also need to celebrate in its fierceness. Just because we name and know ourselves as resilient does not mean we are perfect. It also does not mean we are damaged. This mantle of resilience is the armor for battles and warmth during colder times. It is the quality that allows us to hold others and the reminder that sometimes we need to be held.

The Problem of Resilience

Some might say we should not need to be resilient. We should not need to feel as though we need to go back to a certain place in order to be okay, to move on. This conversation seems to assume there is one definition of resilience for everyone. It assumes there is one place we are supposed to head to once the trouble is over and things are not immediately dangerous. And everyone should go there and be there -- and then everything is okay.

No. To seek out resilience is not an act of seeking out a certain state of being. It is the act of strengthening a muscle that will hold us up when all else falls around us. Cultivating resilience is the promise to ourselves that we will be okay and that we are held in our not-okayness. Like a daily practice, we can come back to this place of knowing and being. Because we have set up the space for it to be present. Because we know we will wander away from thinking we can handle things. We might wander so far away that we forget where we started in the first place. But we can come back.

Should the world create situations in which we must be resilient? Should some be in families that were so harmful that resilience became as vital as breathing? Should we have to face the worst possible situations in order to know we are okay despite everything burning around us? I'm not sure anyone can answer those questions. I know I'd rather have a world that allows us to have more joy than pain, and this is mostly my experience. While I might not remember this when the pain is really painful, I also know its presence allows me to know joy more intimately.

When my mom was killed in a car accident, I remember telling someone that it was a very horrible and very beautiful time. Things became clearer than they had been before. I didn't hide behind what I thought I should feel. I felt it all. I felt it out loud and dramatically. And sometimes, I didn't feel anything. I didn't say anything. Some days, I didn't think I was strong enough to bear it. Some days, I really wished I was with my mom instead of feeling the pain I felt. But, with practices that supported my body, mind, and spirit, I came back. It was not an overnight process. It took three years. Three years. But I came back stronger, wiser. I returned not to the place I 'should' be, but to the place of the new me that I had become -- or perhaps that had been revealed as the true me.

I'm not sure what the transformation was, as there are ways I don't recognize myself today and there are ways that I am proud of the person I am now, and the way that I am more alive because of death. If there was ever a moment when I knew my resilience, it was the moment I came home from the funeral and realized my life would never be the same. And while it would be many months until I could hold onto the knowledge of my resilience, I took a breath and knew I would get through it. Even if 'getting through it' was the best I could do. Sometimes, it is.

I want to be clear that cultivating resilience does not need to come from a horrible place. It can come from simply wanting to be ready for things that knock you off balance. You can be ready for all that life can offer -- good and bad. To be sure, some good things have knocked me off my center too and I used my resilience there too. Perhaps it's not about the instigating event, but about the desire to bring into ourselves the power of deep trust and knowing. When we can trust ourselves in the shadows of our life, we can live in the sunlight more openly and with gratitude.

Fight / Flight / Freeze / Fawn

It can help to understand why we are acting the way we are acting. This allows us to better know and appreciate our responses as being normal versus being a sign that we are damaged. While there are thoughts about how early life experiences impact the way we attach to others and thus the way we attach to people throughout our lives, we are going to stick with the most relevant topic to resilience -- your response to perceived danger.

Our bodies are hardwired to keep us safe. We are designed to do whatever it takes to stay alive, even when it doesn't make a lot of sense when we're out of that danger zone. For example, when we believe we are being attacked by someone else, we might run away immediately because that puts the most space between our bodies and the potential for harm. Or we may have learned that playing nice is the way to make sure we're not hurt. Or something else. All of this is a normal response and reaction to what might hurt us. However, we can also look for new ways to respond -- perhaps healthier and more effective responses.

When we perceive a threat, our bodies will begin to take action. We begin to make more adrenaline that will power us in any decision we make about our safety. This adrenaline allows us to have more power and it also signals to the rest of the body that non-essential tasks need to stop. We can react in a few different ways when we perceive danger. Often, this is referred to as the fight or flight response, but there are actually many more responses we can have. Let's look at the ways in which you are most likely to respond in times of danger:

Fight - For some, the first reaction will be to fight back against the threat. This is the way to stop the harm and it can also help you feel more in control of the situation. More often than not, people will do this when they feel their life is in immediate danger, not even thinking about the potential harm this action might cause on them or another.
Flight - And for others, there is a possibility that one might run away from a problem when it arises. They might run away from the threat literally, or they might distance themselves in another way. For many who are unable to think of another way to respond, running away can be the first thought.

But there are two others responses that are most often discussed in relationship to resilience: freeze and fawn.

Freeze - If you've ever seen or heard of an opossum, you know the freeze response. When you are in a situation that is completely terrifying, real or imagined, you might simply freeze. This often shows up in stories of abuse when people simply 'left their bodies' while the event was happening while their bodies remained.
Fawn - This reaction is slightly newer in conversations as it's a little less recognizable as a response. If you are a person who enters a dangerous situation and immediately tries to make everything okay or to reduce the intensity of the situation, you might be someone whose response is to fawn. People who have been in abusive situations will often let their abuser know that everything is okay, as they don't want to excite them any further.

It's important to look at these responses not just in the landscape of harm, but also in the context of interactions with others. If you're exposed to a scary situation, notice how you respond. You don't have to change anything right now, but this response can help you see what you are doing and what you might be able to do differently. (Of course, when you're in actual physical and emotional danger, do whatever you can to get away. No matter if it makes sense. It will save you.)

- When you notice you are fighting, you might decide to take a breath before responding.
- When you notice you are fleeing, you might remind yourself you are safe and to stay in the situation to see it through.
- When you notice you are freezing, take a moment to come back into your body so you can be present and grounded.
- When you notice you are fawning, you can come back to your body to ask what is important to you. When you can tap back into the truth of your body and experience, you can be fully engaged and in your power.

Resilience is born out of our reactions and born out of learning how we respond when things get difficult. The more we know about how we act, the more we can begin to take action and to take control of those reactions. But trauma has an impact. And often our responses are etched into our bodies when we have faced hard and horrible things. (And before you discount your own life as being trauma-free, nearly everyone has encountered some level of trauma. It's common to the human experience. It's not a sign of damage. It's a sign that something happened that hurt you. Learning more can help you use your lessons and leverage them into wisdom.)

The Impact of Trauma

Because resilience is so often connected with traumatic events, this is often the place to begin learning about this practice of coming back. The body has a number of interesting reactions to traumatic events and building resilience before those events begin can help soften the blows of the inevitable.

Trauma is a situation in which something unexpected happens, causing physical or emotional harm, causing distress. For those who are more resilient and possibly more exposed to trauma, these situations are bumps on the road versus obstacles. For those who have not had a lot of exposure to traumatic events or those who have had constant traumas, resilience is harder won. Traumas might occur due to exposure to:

- Wartime / battle / life-threatening situations
- Natural disasters / manmade disasters
- Rape / incest / torture / neglect / abuse
- Repeated exposure to unsafe conditions
- Accidents / deaths / illnesses
- Intrusive medical procedures
- Breakups / divorces / parental separation
- Ongoing stressors
- One-time stressors

But while this is a short list, it does not encompass what can be traumatic to many people. While it might be one thing to say that certain things are likely to cause trauma, it is another thing to say that only certain things are traumatizing.

After all, you might be more prone to being traumatized by seeing a car accident after you know someone who has been in one or you have been in one. While someone else who has not been exposed to a car accident before may not be traumatized by seeing one happen. There is no right or wrong way to do trauma. There is only the impact of a situation and how it caused trauma.

Trauma often shows up as (per HelpGuide.org):

- Shock, denial, or disbelief
- Confusion, difficulty concentrating
- Anger, irritability, mood swings
- Anxiety and fear
- Guilt, shame, self-blame
- Withdrawing from others
- Feeling sad or hopeless
- Feeling disconnected or numb
- Insomnia or nightmares
- Fatigue
- Being startled easily
- Difficulty concentrating
- Racing heartbeat
- Edginess and agitation
- Aches and pains
- Muscle tension

Trauma often shows up as physical or emotional symptoms we quickly attribute to something else. In a society that can often seem to believe that bleeding is the only kind of trauma, we are very quick to dismiss what we feel as trauma -- and to dismiss what we've experienced as trauma. After all, if we are still alive and we are safe, things must be just fine, right? But trauma arrives as it does for any number of reasons. It might show up immediately or years later -- or not at all. Trauma can be stuffed back, hidden, and ignored. Or it can be all-consuming and unmanageable.

Most often, trauma is something that needs to be managed and supported by a qualified mental health professional. In situations of extreme and ongoing trauma, a therapist or counselor can offer tools to bring you relief and safety. There are also tools you can use on your own to help you begin to heal and to activate your resilience.

Safe space - This has been called multiple things depending on the practitioner and the practice. In some traditions of witchcraft, it is also known as a place of power or a place that a trance might occur. When you create a safe space, you call into your mind a place where you feel completely at ease. This might be a beach or a cottage in the woods or a mountain. You call into your mind this space so clearly that you can feel it and experience it. This is the place where you want to return when things get too activated in your life. For example, when you experience tough emotions about a trauma, you can return to this safe space to calm down. It's like an escape plan where you can restore yourself until you feel ready to take on more emotions and more experience. The more you work with this safe space, the more you will be able to call the feeling it conjures into your mind and body. And the more you can do this, the more resilience you can cultivate in your life.

TRE - When animals are in the wild and they are in danger, they will often play dead and freeze. This causes the predator to often leave them alone. But when the predator leaves, the animal that was being pursued will then get up and continue to shake or run as they were before they froze. The animal seeks to complete the cycle in order to release the stress hormones from their body. We humans don't do that. We might freeze or flee, but we typically don't finish the cycle, causing us to store stress in our bodies. Instead, we could use a practice like TRE (Trauma Releasing Exercises) to help move trauma out of the body. While there are classes and videos online to help walk you through the practice, you can do something simple at home -- shake. Just try to shake your body at the end of the day until you feel stress and tension leave your body. Or you can walk or dance or move in some

way to bring your body back to the present moment.
Hug yourself - Another way to bring your body back to itself and to calm yourself is to hug yourself. Cross your arms over the front of your body and hug yourself with one hand over the opposite shoulder and one hand over the other shoulder. This is meant to sync the two sides of your body with the two sides of your brain. When you do this, you will calm everything down. This will help you release trauma and while the memory will still be there, it will also be less activating to you in the present moment.
Presence your body - One of the experts in trauma and attending to trauma is Peter Levine. He offers a practice of coming back to your body as often as possible. Because trauma often requires us to leave our bodies (either physically or emotionally), we need to learn how to come back in order to heal and to be fully alive. An exercise that he offers is to use the shower to come back to the physical experience of yourself. You can place a part of your body in the water's stream and name that part of your body. You might say, "This is my hand. This is the hand of my body." You can repeat this again and again until you begin to feel that you are in your body.

One way I have used this practice in classes about coming back to the body is to find a partner, someone you trust or someone you could imagine trusting in this exercise. Stand across from your partner and allow yourself to find places of your body that hold the stories of trauma. You don't have to think of the most traumatic events in your life, nor do you need to presence every trauma you've ever experienced. Instead, think of a few and sense where they live in your body. Is there tension in your neck? In your shoulders? In your stomach? When you have located these areas, touch them and have your partner silently witness the introduction to your stories of trauma. If you are sharing, you might use the words, "This is my neck. This is the neck of my body."

Continue this sharing until you feel that you have presenced what you want to presence. Once you have, then you can switch roles with your partner and have them share. At the end, you might want to hug, if that feels good, or you might want to sit in silence, journal, or simply express emotions that have arisen. The thought behind this practice is that the more you come back to your body, the easier it will be. Instead of leaving the body and thinking it's not safe to be in your body, you can come back to yourself, love yourself, and be grounded where you are.

* * *

All of these practices (and many others!) are not designed to get rid of the trauma. You are never going to get rid of what happened to you or around you. Instead, you can cultivate resilience to allow you to better respond to those events. While you could be stuck and angry at the world for something that happened to you (and for all the right reasons), you can also work to not be angry at those who did not have a role in the situation.

You can learn how to respond effectively in situations that require your response, but not your reaction. You can release the trauma from your body so it doesn't creep up and cause other issues in your life. What has happened to you is not your fault AT ALL. And if you want to move forward in your life in a new way, it can help to build up resources and tools for managing the trauma you do have in your somatic (body) experience.

Talking to Yourself

If you have begun to look at ways to become more resilient and to face your trauma, you might find the practice of positive self-talk to be a common bit of advice. This is not about necessarily cultivating optimism, but rather finding ways to reframe the feelings you might be having. In doing so, you can become your own cheerleader and ally. You can become a person you can rely on for strength.

If you're not used to talking positively to yourself, you're not alone. Many people are not given this skill by their friends and family as it can seem selfish or even narcissistic to feel good about yourself. Let's let that idea go. You have every right to feel good about yourself and to want good things for yourself.

To become your own ally, it can help in times when you are not struggling to write things down that you appreciate about yourself. Think about things you know you do well and things you have accomplished in the past. You can also write down how you have approached difficult times in the past. What did you do? How did you surprise yourself? How strong were you?

When you create these love letters to yourself, you will create a repository of reminders when you need them. If you find yourself in a place where you are down and unmotivated or you just don't believe in yourself, come back to these stories. Pick a few affirmations that allow you to come back to the truth of who you are and who you already have been. After all, when you've made it to this point, you've already made it through the toughest day of your life. And survived.

I am strong.
I am steady and sure.
I am grounded in myself.
I trust that I will know what to do next.
I trust the universe to hold me and guide me.
I am calm and collected.
I am wise and ready for whatever might come.
I have already faced impossible things.
I can make hard decisions.
I am loved and supported.

It is best to use phrases that talk in the present tense and in the 'I am' rather than 'I am becoming' since you want to remind yourself that you already are these things. Perhaps you just need to be reminded a bit more. Some of these phrases may not be easy to say to yourself. But the more you do, the more you will be able to believe them to be true. I encourage you to choose one of these or something else to repeat to yourself over the course of a day. Write it down on a mirror, on a piece of paper, in your wallet, or on your skin under your clothes. Try to take it into your body as a promise and a prayer to your sacred self. Take in the energy of what you already are and the resilience you already embody.

Some find it helpful to have a symbol of this strength somewhere in their living space. Or you might have a piece of jewelry that reminds you. Or you might decide to whisper these prayers into your water bottle or coffee or tea and then drink it in. You can find a ritual that works for you and that works to help you become fully embodied in your brilliant self.

Find Your Priorities

Building your resilience takes practice and takes focused effort. And it can be hard to figure out what to do next when everything and everyone around you seems to be important. But not everything is as important all the time. You might realize as you are moving through this chapter or this entire book that you have not made yourself a priority. You may have begun to realize that you allow others to take up your brain space and your energy. And while this is done to help others, it doesn't always leave a lot of space for you.

So, it's time to name things as priorities in your life. Not only will this help you get to the places you want to go, but it will also help you understand when you need to take action -- and when you do not. You can think to yourself: is this a priority? If so, act. If it's not a priority, you can get to that when you get to it.

Think for yourself right now what your priorities are. Are they things you want to achieve? Are these priorities people you want to connect with? What do you feel is most important to you right now? This is a time when you need to be honest with yourself about yourself. Let go of what others think of your priorities. Instead, think about what you want to bring into your life, where you want to put your energy.

Your physical health
Your emotional health
Your financial health
Your safety
Your family life
Your children

To be clear, there will likely be things that emerge as priorities on certain days. (For example, if you have a sick kid and you're the only caregiver, you may need to put your needs to the side for a moment. Or you might think about how you can get help the next time so you're not always putting your needs aside.) What do really want to focus on right now? If you're not sure what to say, then think about how you want to feel in your life. Once you have those feelings in a list, stop and think about what would make you feel those feelings. (Now, you may find out that things are a bit more complicated than that, but this is a good exercise of learning more about yourself.) Once you have a clearer picture of the why, you can begin to see the 'how' and the things that are most important to you right now.

Write it down.
Write them all down.
Claim them to be yours.

Find ways to focus on each of these dreams and goals every day.

When you do, you will be living a life that feels good and one that allows you to face difficult things. When you already have a softer foundation and a supportive life, harder situations and experiences are less challenging. There will be situations that might seem overwhelming but you will be able to come back more easily.

Resourcing

It's more common to think about resources when our resources are too low -- and we finally realize we're scraping the bottom of our cup. But resourcing can start anytime, even now. You can stockpile the things you need for the times you really need them. What you might need to be resilient may differ from others, and they can still be exactly what you need.

Resourcing is about creating internal and external systems of support. These support systems will allow you to have something to draw upon when things are hard. You will not be alone in your life. You will be able to turn to someone, something, or to yourself to have what you need when you need it.

The upside of resourcing is not only avoiding rock bottom in your life, but also maintaining hope in dark times. When you know you have things to help, you can remember that, in time, you will feel better and things will be better than they are in the present moment. Resourcing can look like:

- Naming feelings
- Tracking feelings and emotions
- Slowing things down
- Welcoming what is
- Being compassionate to yourself

When you're in a difficult situation or you're trying to deal with a difficult problem, it is wise to name the feelings you have. This will help you to see them as being things that are happening and things that are true in the moment. What is the emotion I'm having? It is said there are 10 basic human emotions:

- Joy
- Excitement
- Surprise
- Sadness
- Anger
- Disgust
- Contempt
- Fear
- Shame
- Guilt

Of these feelings, what is present right now? What does your body have to tell you? What feelings are arising? Try to practice not attaching judgment or meaning to these feelings. Simply let them be observations that are happening. From there, you can begin to look at where those feelings seem to be in your body. You might take a bath or go on a walk and simply follow the sensations that arise. Tension? Softness? Do the feelings travel from one place of your body to the next?

It can help to state what you are experiencing out loud. You don't have to do this in front of people, but when you can act like an observer, this will help you clearly understand what is happening. And when you can put a name to it, the feeling becomes less unmanageable. The feeling becomes something you can look at and not be the victim of.

If it's at all possible, try to slow things down in your body and in your mind. This can be accomplished as going back to your breath, slowing it down until it is something that fills you with ease. You can use slow inhalations and long exhalations to not only come back to your body, but also to decrease your heart rate. When you do this, you allow your body to remember that it's not in danger. It does not need to prepare to fight, flight, freeze, or fawn. Calm the body by breathing slowly and steadily. You might also want to try breathing in through your nose and out through your mouth until you feel calmer.

One of the things that seems simple, but can be profound is welcoming what is happening to yourself. The first thing we often want to do when things are hard is deny they are happening or to try to prevent them from taking up too much of our awareness. But when we push things away for too long, we can create ideal circumstances for the feelings to come back even more forcefully -- and unexpectedly. Instead, I invite you to try to welcome all of your feelings as being messengers. They are delivering notes to you about what is going on in your life. They are not harmful, nor are they instructions. They are just information.

Along with this practice of welcoming what is, offer to yourself some compassion and love for your situation. You don't need to fix yourself or be anything more than you are right now. You can just be compassionate toward the you that is going through something hard. The more you come back to your resourcing skills, the more you will be able to create a response that looks like softer concern and care versus rigid reaction.

Inner Allies

While there are many practitioners that offer guidance on how to cultivate inner allies, I found Laurel Parnell to be the most influential for me. In her work with trauma and with building resilience, she offers the simple practice of tapping your body to 'install' resources. This might look like resources that are your safe space or that are people who you admire. Or you might choose to work with a deity or with some other spiritual ally. (I personally have certain allies that I call upon for different resources. For example, I might call on Hecate when I want support during a difficult decision. Or I might call on Aphrodite when I want to call in more love.)

You can choose allies that are in your real life or they can be allies you create to help you when you need them. You might want to start with something you can easily picture in your mind. This might be a being you admire, like Wonder Woman. Her energy might be just what you need when you are feeling powerless.

To 'install' this ally, you just need to sit in a way that is comfortable for you. Get grounded and present and calm. Close your eyes or soften your gaze to allow yourself to become aware of your body's sensations. Bring the picture of Wonder Woman (or whomever you choose) into your mind. What is she like? What powers does she embody? What do you admire about her? Bring up all of these answers and feelings into your body, and as you do, start to tap one side of your body with one hand, then the other, and repeat. Tap your knees or thighs again and again as you feel your body connect with your thoughts. The rhythm should be one, two, one, two, no faster and no slower.

At a certain point, you are likely to feel yourself become calm and steady. When you feel that, you can stop and come back to the room. If you find your thoughts wandering or you don't feel relaxed, continue to think about the positive qualities of Wonder Woman (or whomever you choose) until you start to feel connected and calm.

If your thoughts wander into negative feelings, stop tapping and come back to simply breathing. Once you can return to the positive thoughts, you can begin to tap again. This practice allows you to wire into your body the sensation of an ally. You might find you can call up this image of the ally in your head -- and immediately feel calm.

Feel free to repeat this practice as long as it serves you. You might also choose to have several allies that can be called on in different situations. They can be alive, dead, fictional, etc. They're YOUR allies. The more allies you have around you, the more resilient you can be.

* * *

With all of the talk around resilience today, it's clear that society recognizes that we need more than just to 'get through.' We need to ready ourselves before we enter the shadows of our lives. We need to have the resources in hand to show us the way and to catch us when the danger has passed. From there, we can be allies for others, for ourselves, and for the life that wants us to enjoy it fully.

Tools to Maintain Your Energy

During your journey, you may have noticed the ways your energy has changed and shifted. You might have days when things feel like they are moving in the right direction and other days when things don't feel they're moving in the right direction. You might have times when you have all the energy in the world -- and times when you feel your energy is lagging. To help you maintain your energy and your focus, you can practice a few different exercises to cultivate awareness of yourself.

Knowing Your Size

You can do this practice alone or with a partner. Start with yourself and feeling into the way you feel about yourself right now. Stop and think about what it would feel like if you were a person who never felt like they did anything wrong. They were always right and they were always perfect. Imagine yourself as a know-it-all, over-confident person. Inflated.

What does that feel like in your body?
What does that feel like in your mind?

From there, shake off that feeling and come back to your body as it is when you feel confident in the world. Come back to the right size of your being, the one that knows how to connect with others and the one that feels comfortable. Right sized. Think about a time when you were completely yourself. Let that fill you and move you in the space.

What does that feel like in your body?
What does that feel like in your mind?

Shake that feeling off and allow yourself to bring into your body the feeling of being deflated and depressed. Think about how it feels when you don't think you're worth anything. Think about how it feels when you are sad and alone and worried that you will never figure things out. Think about how it feels when the world is crashing around you and you're pretty sure it's all your fault.

What does that feel like in your body?
What does that feel like in your mind?

Shake that off. Allow yourself to come back to the right size of yourself. This practice allows you to see where your energy is in this moment. Sometimes, you might feel bigger or smaller than your normal self. But in this practice, you can also get better at moving between states of being.

When you feel your energy is starting to get too big, what can you do to come back to your right sized self? When you feel your energy too low, what can you do to move it to a more grounded state? Again, this takes practice and a willingness to feel as though you're making things up. It also takes practice to not believe there is only one way to feel or be in the world. All of us are deflated at times, inflated at others, and right sized at others. And some of us are much more comfortable in the deflated. Or the inflated. By knowing this, we can see when we need to do things to bring ourselves back to the place we want to be.

Running Energy in Your Body

A practice in some witchcraft and magical traditions is to run energy through the body as though the body were a star or pentacle. There are many different possibilities for this and there are many different pentacles that you might use or create.

This tool can be used to help you move certain energies into your body or it can be used to help you diagnose where issues live in your body. For example, if you run energy and you find it feels stuck in one area, you might look at the energy that area holds. How can you balance this in your life? How can you bring more attention to it? How can you look at this area in a new way?

The basic movement of energy in the body looks like this:

Start with bringing your awareness in a ball that settles at the top of your head. Focus on the energy of that place. What lives there? What is known and unknown here?

Move the energy down your body to your right foot and the next energy point. What lives here? What is known and unknown here?

From there, move the energy up the body and over to the left hand and that energy point. What lives here? What is known and unknown here?

From the left hand, move across the body to the right hand and that place of energy. What lives here? What is known and unknown here?

Moving back down the body, travel to the left foot and that point of energy. What lives here? What is known and unknown here?

And return to the top of the head.

You can repeat these movements, always ending with the top of the head.

You can also choose to close the pentacle by moving from the top of the head to the left hand to the left foot to the right foot to the right hand and back to the top of the head.

In doing this, you may choose to stand with your legs spread out a little further than shoulder width and your arms stretched out in a straight line, parallel to the floor. Or you might choose to hold your body in a comfortable way that works for your body. You can stand up, lie down, or find another way to run this energy. Some of the pentacles you can use include:

- Iron - Sex, Pride, Self, Power, Passion
- Pearl - Love, Law, Knowledge, Liberation, Wisdom
- Blessing - Devotion, Truth, Radiance, Grace, Blessing
- Devotion, Compassion, Acceptance, Connection, Ecstasy
- Spirit, Water, Air, Earth, Fire

You can also choose to use other words and energies that make more sense to you. The point is to make sure you are running energies that help to ground you. When you notice things are out of sync or things feel sticky or strange, it's best to look at how those energies are being tended to in your life. Or not. You can also continue to run the energies until you feel they are back in your body. You can also send extra attention and energy to those places as you run the pentacles. The more you use this tool of earth, the more you can come into awareness of yourself and your experience. And when you have more awareness, you free up energy that was lost in confusion or speculation.

Grounding, Always

To bring back your energy, go back to the source of energy -- the Earth. I often say to students that when you're working with magick, the energy you use should not be solely your own. You should be tapping into the energy of the Earth. By taking time to ground down and to reach up to the sky, you allow yourself to be the conduit between these two places. You can always stretch down and stretch up to find the energy you need.

One time, I was feeling very tired at a large pagan event. It was the first time I'd ever been and I was not prepared for the energy swirling around me. I thought I hadn't gotten enough sleep or that I'd eaten too much sugar, and that was the reason for my tiredness. But someone came up to me and asked if I had grounded yet that day. I realized I had been using all of my own energy to sustain myself. Instead, I could have called on the Earth to help and to hold.

No matter what you do for grounding, no matter if you follow the various instructions in this book or you find another way to tap back into the ground beneath you, this is the place for restoration and energy. The Earth always has what you need.

* * *

While you have already learned a lot of tools for running energy and tracking energy, you also want to watch your energy to see when it needs help. Allow yourself to be the protector of your energetic inventory. Ask for what you need, run the energy of the Earth, and take rest when you need rest. This work of being healthy and well requires energy -- and a new relationship to our energy. And we don't do this work alone.

Support Systems No Matter What

Humans are hardwired for connection, it is said. And while we might know that being with others will feel better and more grounding, we might still have moments where we just want to be alone. One of my favorite coping mechanisms is to move away from other people as much as possible, returning only when I feel I've put myself back together again. Not only does this mean I end up facing things alone, but it also means that I don't have the connection with people who love me and support me. Setting up support systems was one of the best things I did for myself, but I only learned of their importance once I looked back on how things could have been.

Know What You Need

Sometimes, it's not that we don't have the support we need, but rather that we don't know how to tell others what we need. It seems like people who love us should just know what we need -- and sometimes this is true -- but more often than not, they wait for us to tell them what to do. So, we need to know what we need when things are hard.

Communication - Do you need to have someone call you or try to call you? Do you want someone to text you without any expectation of response? Do you want to talk to someone every day, at odd hours of the day, etc.? What kind of communication do you need?

Contact - Do you want to be touched when you are feeling down? Do you want someone to be in the same room as you but not touch you? Do you want someone to hold you for long periods or short periods? Do you need someone to ask you about touch before they touch you?

Love language - While some might think love languages are

only for couples, they can also help us in other relationships. Created by Gary Chapman, love languages include: Words of Affirmation; Gifts; Acts of Service; Quality Time; and Physical Touch. Which of these help you feel loved? You may have more than one that helps you feel loved, and that's okay. Being able to clearly state that something makes you feel loved can help someone else show up for you in a way that has meaning.

I often describe this process of teaching someone how to love you and to support you as creating a Care and Feeding of YOUR NAME manual.

You could create this when you're not in crisis. It should be something you send to everyone who loves you and who wants to support you. You can adjust it as you learn more about yourself, of course, but this list would be great to have on hand as a starting point so you don't have to start from nothing when you're already feeling depleted.

Know Who Loves You

Right now, not later, write down a list of people who care about you. Write down a list of people who love you and who have been there for you when things have been tough. Take your time to list every single person that loves you. From that list, look at the people who are there. Think about how they have enriched your life. Consider how they have told you that they love you and how they have showed you that they love you.

Make this list something you can look at whenever you might need to remember others. Make this list because these are the people you need to communicate with about your needs and desires during tough times. Sometimes, just knowing there are people out in the world that love you can help bring you out of a dark state of being. Sometimes, knowing you are loved can help you when you feel you are unlovable.

Set up Systems of Support

With the list of how to care for you when things are down and a list of people to reach out to, you also need to take action. If no one knows you are suffering, they will not know you need help. So many people in the United States, especially, have been brought up to live in a mindset of 'rugged individualism' in which we are taught we need to do everything on our own. We need to suffer through and not ask for help because asking for help means we are weak. It's time to let that idea die.

We all need help from time to time, even the ones who seem to have everything together. We all have moments when we don't know what to do or where to go with our problems. We all need someone sometimes. No one person has all the answers and no one person should be expected to. It can help today or in a moment where you're not overwhelmed by life to figure out what you will do when you begin to feel that you need more support in your life. A few ideas might look like:

Set up regular friend dates - It can help to have ongoing dates with friends to stay connected at all times. This doesn't have to be more than a quick weekly phone call or email, or it could mean that you all meet somewhere to grab coffee. The more you can get out and be in contact, the more you may be able to avoid the feelings of isolation before they become too challenging.

Have a signal for trouble - When you realize you need support, whatever that looks like to you, you may want to agree to a certain signal that will let the other person know things are hard. For example, some people like to use text messaging to send a certain emoji or phrase that quickly lets the other person know they need help.

Ask for what you think you need - Though it might be hard,

asking for what you need is the best way to get what you need. Even if you double-guess yourself along the way, try asking for something and allowing yourself to receive it. While you might find the request doesn't make you feel as good as you hoped it would, knowing someone is there can still be supportive.

Reach out to multiple people - If you are facing a difficult situation and you need support from others, it is best to reach out to multiple people at the same time. Though it might seem as though you don't need everyone to answer, the more support you have, the better. It's always great to have more people watching out for you than fewer.

This is not a practice that comes easily to everyone. It might feel like work to ask for help and to be clear with others about what you need. It might feel uncomfortable, needy, and self-serving. And maybe it is. So what? It's okay to be uncomfortable once in a while. It shows us where we are growing and learning. It's okay to be needy because sometimes we need more than we have. It's okay to serve yourself because you are worthy of attention and care.

Self-Support Strategies

And it should be said that there will be moments when people you love can't be there for you. They might be going through a difficult period too or they might not be able to give you the energy and attention you need. For someone who may not be comfortable asking for support, it can be hard to hear that you don't have the support you expected. (Chances are good you will find what you need, but it's also good to be prepared.) When this happens, you need to return to the inner structures of support you have created for yourself. You can also do things to reduce the discomfort you feel when things are hard:

Ground - Come back to your body. Imagine roots into the earth and branches up to the sky. Know yourself as the kiss between earth and heaven.

Return to your safe space - Return to the place that you know to be safe in your mind. When things are feeling unsteady, perhaps make this space better, prettier, more vibrant in your mind.

Take 90 seconds - Some research has shown that it takes about 90 seconds for the mind to experience an emotion. If you can wait out that time period, you can come back to a less emotional state from which you can solve problems and look at things more clearly.

Move your body - When you are feeling overwhelmed and stuck, try to move your body in some way. This allows you to create momentum, even if it doesn't change anything about the situation.

Sing / scream - Getting your voice opened up will help you feel more in alignment with your body. When you bring yourself back to your voice, you become present with what you're doing and saying and how you sound. This can bring you back to calm.

And sometimes, you might just need to have moments when things feel overwhelming. This is NORMAL. This is human. More often than not, the feelings will pass. The feelings will settle. You will settle. You will figure out what to do next or the next steps will reveal themselves.

* * *

Support can arrive in many different ways. It can show up as a person, as a promise, or as the passage of time. When you know what you need and who loves you, you will be able to feel less alone and worried in the world. You need people. And people need you. The more you can know and get what you need, the more grounded you will become. And when you're more grounded, you can help others return to themselves too.

Conclusion

The journey to health and wellness begins when it begins. In fact, it has already begun with the attention you've given and offered. No matter your intention right now and no matter the goals you have for your life, your health and well-being are in your hands. You can start where you are, with the things you already have, and create a life that supports the wondrousness of you.

I invite you to the blessing that you can be to your own life. With presence and practice, you can step onto a path that allows you to be fully imperfect and engaged in the present moment. And you've already shown up. You've already begun. With your presence, your creativity, your wisdom, your breath, and your being, you can build the foundation. You can make your vessel strong and your spirit vibrant. You can meet the divine in the promises you make and the chances you take to care for yourself so deeply that nothing can shake you.

While balance might be impossible and self-care a bit more boring than it's been advertised, you are equipped with the tools of your unfolding. You are ready to open up to a life that offers excitement and challenge, but also resilience. No matter your story and your traumas, you can call up the energy of possibility. You can call on others and on yourself to be fully immersed in this strange journey of being alive. I wish for you all of the wonder and awe that comes with stepping fully into this moment. This precious moment.

When we arrive as we are, when we remember, 'No matter where you go, there you are,' we can bring ourselves back to ourselves. We can remember the value of our being, the strength of ourselves, and the power of speaking up for our needs.

Not everyone will understand. Not everyone will appreciate your new priorities. You will likely face some people who simply do not want you to change. To them, you need to say, you are more important. To the voices inside your head that feel you are asking for too much, you need to quiet them too.

Get quiet. Get present. Get clear.
This journey is one that was made for you.
You precious moment.
You wondrous being.
May you be blessed in your uncovering.
May you be witnessed in your unfolding.
May you be inspired by your own daring.
May you continue to hold yourself well.
Blessed be.

Resources

Books

"Healing Trauma" by Peter Levine, PhD
"Waking the Tiger: Healing Trauma" by Peter Levine, PhD
"Tapping In" by Laurel Parnell, PhD
"The DustBunnies' Big Damn Handout Book" by Valerie Walker (veedub)

Online Resources

90 Second Rule:

https://www.surreymindfulness.co.uk/the-90-second-rule

Pentacles:

http://notesofaferitrainee.blogspot.com/2009/12/four-pentacles-on-tree.html

Resilience:

https://hbr.org/2016/06/resilience-is-about-how-you-recharge-not-how-you-endure?fbclid=IwAR02LhoSnA4OQAZ_2BkGcrP-Koy3mOdrTJmHhKCHuieAi7tLa4nzQ82BPq4

https://www.nytimes.com/2017/07/25/well/mind/how-to-boost-resilience-in-midlife.html?rref=collection%2Fsectioncollection%2Fwell&action=click&contentCollection=well&region=rank&module=package&version=highlights&contentPlacement=1&pgtype=sectionfront

http://www.new-synapse.com/aps/wordpress/?p=1825

Resourcing:

http://relational-integrative-psychotherapy.uk/chapters/resourcing-nurturing-skills-and-mobilising-coping-strategies/

Self-Care:

https://www.outofthestorm.website/self-care

https://www.nytimes.com/interactive/2018/08/11/style/how-i-self-care.html

Trauma:

https://www.helpguide.org/articles/ptsd-trauma/coping-with-emotional-and-psychological-trauma.htm

https://drarielleschwartz.com/complex-ptsd-and-attachment-trauma-dr-arielle-schwartz/?fbclid=IwAR0zRBHf4NT4XbPvGy1fWo320t0b-yMrb5YMo44Wt0b_X2u1tsW4lidqpo0#.XcTJyiVlCEc

https://letsqueerthingsup.com/2019/07/06/7-subtle-signs-your-trauma-response-is-to-fawn/?fbclid=IwAR1QJVDvwvpts2z7wTmEhpe9ArFf8iYoSBwaK6Ub0C_ityyVOFyscOAnU1w

https://traumaprevention.com/

Worksheets / Diagrams

TRACKING MY DAY

WHAT I ATE

HOW IT MADE ME FEEL

HOW I MOVED

HOW IT MADE ME FEEL

HOW I CARED FOR MYSELF

HOW IT MADE ME FEEL

WHAT I BELIEVE AND VALUE

WHAT MY PRIORITIES ARE

THE CARE AND FEEDING OF ______________________

When I feel______________ I need __________________

Things that make me happy

____

____

____

____

____

____

____

Things that distract me

____

____

____

____

____

____

____

Things that help me feel connected

People I trust and love

Foods / Drinks I need

My Love Language

It helps me to hear ....

Create Your Own Pentacle

Here is an image to help you create your own pentacle for running energy.

It might help to print this out or to draw this out on your own so you can create multiple pentacles for your use. You can draw this as the top of the head being the top of the star and the left bottom point as the right foot. Said another way, you can draw your pentacle with the image of your body lying on top of it. (Or do it any way you wish. It's your pentacle!)

MOON
BOOKS

PAGANISM & SHAMANISM

What is Paganism? A religion, a spirituality, an alternative belief system, nature worship? You can find support for all these definitions (and many more) in dictionaries, encyclopaedias, and text books of religion, but subscribe to any one and the truth will evade you. Above all Paganism is a creative pursuit, an encounter with reality, an exploration of meaning and an expression of the soul. Druids, Heathens, Wiccans and others, all contribute their insights and literary riches to the Pagan tradition. Moon Books invites you to begin or to deepen your own encounter, right here, right now.

If you have enjoyed this book, why not tell other readers by posting a review on your preferred book site.

Recent bestsellers from Moon Books are:

Journey to the Dark Goddess
How to Return to Your Soul
Jane Meredith
Discover the powerful secrets of the Dark Goddess and transform your depression, grief and pain into healing and integration.
Paperback: 978-1-84694-677-6 ebook: 978-1-78099-223-5

Shamanic Reiki
Expanded Ways of Working with Universal Life Force Energy
Llyn Roberts, Robert Levy
Shamanism and Reiki are each powerful ways of healing; together, their power multiplies. *Shamanic Reiki* introduces techniques to help healers and Reiki practitioners tap ancient healing wisdom.
Paperback: 978-1-84694-037-8 ebook: 978-1-84694-650-9

Pagan Portals – The Awen Alone
Walking the Path of the Solitary Druid
Joanna van der Hoeven
An introductory guide for the solitary Druid, *The Awen Alone* will accompany you as you explore, and seek out your own place within the natural world.
Paperback: 978-1-78279-547-6 ebook: 978-1-78279-546-9

A Kitchen Witch's World of Magical Herbs & Plants
Rachel Patterson
A journey into the magical world of herbs and plants, filled with magical uses, folklore, history and practical magic. By popular writer, blogger and kitchen witch, Tansy Firedragon.
Paperback: 978-1-78279-621-3 ebook: 978-1-78279-620-6

Shaman Pathways – The Druid Shaman

Exploring the Celtic Otherworld

Danu Forest

A practical guide to Celtic shamanism with exercises and techniques as well as traditional lore for exploring the Celtic Otherworld.

Paperback: 978-1-78099-615-8 ebook: 978-1-78099-616-5

Traditional Witchcraft for the Woods and Forests

A Witch's Guide to the Woodland with Guided Meditations and Pathworking

Mélusine Draco

A Witch's guide to walking alone in the woods, with guided meditations and pathworking.

Paperback: 978-1-84694-803-9 ebook: 978-1-84694-804-6

Wild Earth, Wild Soul

A Manual for an Ecstatic Culture

Bill Pfeiffer

Imagine a nature-based culture so alive and so connected, spreading like wildfire. This book is the first flame…

Paperback: 978-1-78099-187-0 ebook: 978-1-78099-188-7

Naming the Goddess

Trevor Greenfield

Naming the Goddess is written by over eighty adherents and scholars of Goddess and Goddess Spirituality.

Paperback: 978-1-78279-476-9 ebook: 978-1-78279-475-2

Shapeshifting into Higher Consciousness
Heal and Transform Yourself and Our World with Ancient Shamanic and Modern Methods
Llyn Roberts
Ancient and modern methods that you can use every day to transform yourself and make a positive difference in the world.
Paperback: 978-1-84694-843-5 ebook: 978-1-84694-844-2

Readers of ebooks can buy or view any of these bestsellers by clicking on the live link in the title. Most titles are published in paperback and as an ebook. Paperbacks are available in traditional bookshops. Both print and ebook formats are available online.

Find more titles and sign up to our readers' newsletter at http://www.johnhuntpublishing.com/paganism
Follow us on Facebook at https://www.facebook.com/MoonBooks and Twitter at https://twitter.com/MoonBooksJHP